A qualified exercise teac... ...in the field of diet and fitnes... ...1986 that she discovered ... ...low-fat eating led to a leaner body. Forced on to a low-fat diet as a result of a gall-stone problem, not only did Rosemary avoid major surgery but her previously disproportionately large hips and thighs reduced dramatically in size. After extensive research and trials her *Hip and Thigh Diet* was published in 1988 by Arrow Books. This book and its sequel, *Rosemary Conley's Complete Hip and Thigh Diet*, dominated the bestseller lists for over five years and have sold in excess of two million copies. Subsequent titles, *Hip and Thigh Diet Cookbook*, and *New Hip and Thigh Diet Cookbook* (written with chef and cookery writer Patricia Bourne), *Inch Loss Plan*, *Metabolism Booster Diet* and *Whole Body Programme*, have all been instant number one bestsellers.

Rosemary has travelled the world promoting her books and has made numerous appearances on national and international television and radio. Since 1990 she has presented her own diet and fitness series on network television on both the BBC and ITV. Rosemary has also released many fitness videos with total sales exceeding one million copies.

In 1993 the Rosemary Conley Diet and Fitness Clubs were launched across the United Kingdom. Operating under a franchise system, carefully selected instructors are fully trained to teach the Rosemary Conley philosophy at weekly classes throughout the United Kingdom. It has proved to be the fastest growing franchise operation in the United Kingdom, with classes being extremely popular, fulfilling a need to give additional support to existing followers of Rosemary's diets. It is the first national diet and fitness organisation in operation where only qualified instructors are in operation.

Rosemary lives in Leicestershire with her husband Mike Rimmington with whom she runs Rosemary Conley Enterprises and Rosemary Conley Diet and Fitness Clubs Limited. She has a daughter by her first marriage and they are all committed Christians.

Rosemary Conley's
Beach Body Plan

ARROW

First published in 1994

1 3 5 7 9 10 8 6 4 2

© Rosemary Conley Enterprises 1994

First published in the United Kingdom in 1994
by Arrow Books Limited
Random House, 20 Vauxhall Bridge Road,
London SW1V 2SA

Random House, Australia (Pty) Limited
20 Alfred Street, Milsons Point, Sydney,
New South Wales 2061, Australia

Random House New Zealand Limited
18 Poland Road, Glenfield,
Auckland 10, New Zealand

Random House, South Africa (Pty) Limited
PO Box 337, Bergvlei, South Africa

Random House UK Limited Reg. No. 954009

ISBN 0 09 946551 5

Designed by Roger Walker
Nutritional consultant: Penny J. Hunking

Printed in Great Britain by
Cox & Wyman Ltd, Reading

Contents

Acknowledgements

With the ever increasing demands on my time I become even more grateful to all those who help when the deadline approaches for the manuscript to be delivered. I would like to offer my grateful thanks to Emma Archer, for so patiently beavering away at transforming my scribble and dictation into legible print. Also, to Janet Thomson for hcr help with the design of the exercise section and never-ending pool of knowledge regarding exercise and its benefits. Thanks also to The Potato Marketing Board for contributing many of the recipes included in this book which I have modified to a low-fat formula.

The unsung hero of any book is the editor. I have worked with Jan Bowmer on all of my books since the *Hip and Thigh Diet*. Not only is she a very dear friend but she is very encouraging and extremely supportive as well as possessing a great talent for editing my work into a popular format. Thanks are due also to Dennis Barker, art director, and to Roger Walker, text designer.

WARNING

If you have a medical condition, or are pregnant, the diet and exercises described in this book should not be followed without first consulting your doctor. All guidelines and warnings should be read carefully, and the author and publisher cannot accept responsibility for injuries or damage arising out of a failure to comply with the same.

'A well designed, nutritionally balanced, sensible and satisfying 28–day eating plan to help you get into shape for summer'

Penny J. Hunking, R.S.A., S.R.D., P.E.A.
Dietitian

STAGE I

Getting Started

If you want to look *significantly* slimmer and in much better *shape* for this summer, this 28-day *Beach Body Plan* is for *you*. It's easy, it's effective, it's safe and it's fun. There's plenty to eat so you won't feel as if you are dieting, and the physical activity involved is varied and unregimented. In just four weeks it will make a real difference to how you look when you 'strip off' for the beach!

I am not going to bore you with the physiological facts of how and why we turn excess food into fat or why some people can eat mountains of goodies and stay thin, while others, like me, have to eat carefully and moderately, or run the risk of expanding to the proportions of Billy Bunter! If you've bought this book you are likely to be in the latter category and looking for help – in fact, instant help – to perform a miracle on your body before you embark on your annual trip to the sea and sun. The good news is a *great* deal *can* be achieved in four weeks. If you stick strictly to this *Beach Body Plan*, you will be staggered at the results. But first you must ask yourself the following questions:

	YES	NO
1 Do I really want to lose significant amounts of fat from my body before my holiday?	☐	☐
2 Am I prepared to make some changes/sacrifices to my daily diet over the next four weeks to achieve a leaner body for my holiday?	☐	☐
3 Am I willing to undertake some form of physical activity on five days in each of the four weeks?	☐	☐
4 Am I prepared to ignore *all* foods on the 'forbidden list' for the duration of this plan?	☐	☐
5 When eating out, am I prepared to ask for my food to be cooked and served without fat?	☐	☐
6 Am I prepared to give permission to my family and friends to watch over and reprimand me if necessary?	☐	☐

If you answered 'yes' to all these questions you can look forward to achieving a body of which you can be proud – in just four weeks. *Nobody else* can do this for you. Only *you* can decide what goes into your mouth. Only *you* can make the physical effort to play a game of sport or do an exercise workout at home or at your local gym or class. But it doesn't have to be purgatory. You won't have to go hungry or do any form of exercise you don't enjoy. This is going to be FUN, and at the end of the four weeks you are going to feel FANTASTIC.

STAGE 2

How The Plan Works

Each day of this plan contains two choices of menu for breakfast, lunch and dinner. In addition, an evening snack (treat) is allowed, or this can be taken as a dessert to accompany the evening meal. Throughout the 28 days only the menus included in this book must be used. However, with a total of 56 options for each meal, there is no reason to be bored.

All of the menus have been designed to give optimum nutrition and maximum bulk in order to keep the metabolic rate (the rate at which we burn off calories) buoyant. Each person's metabolic rate responds to the amount of food they eat. If we eat too little it slows down and the body's ability to burn off fat is greatly reduced. This is Nature's way of protecting us against possible future starvation. If the body receives too little nourishment, it compensates by holding on to the small amount of food it *does* receive, converting it to reserves of fat instead of using it for energy. Although, under such circumstances, we would lose weight, we wouldn't lose fat. Instead we would lose water, plus lean body tissue (muscle) – the very part of our body that can help increase our metabolic rate. It's a fact that the greater the amount of muscle mass on our bodies, the higher our metabolic rate. We therefore need to encourage the maintenance of existing muscles and aim to *increase* that muscle mass with strengthening exercises.

The good news is that we *can* keep our metabolic rate buoyant and still lose actual body fat by following two golden rules. First, we should eat regular and normal-sized meals and, second, we should combine this sensible pattern with physical activity. Indeed, through careful lifestyle and body management, we can *increase* our metabolic rate. Let me explain.

A simple way to illustrate how the metabolic rate fluctuates is to imagine a gas flame. If we eat healthily at regular intervals throughout the day and take moderate physical exercise, the metabolic rate burns away quite happily on a medium flame. But if we were to go on a crash diet, skipping meals or eating a 'very low-calorie meal replacement-type' diet, the metabolic rate would reduce to a tiny flame producing minimal heat. This is *just* what the dieter wants to avoid, since it reduces the body's effectiveness at converting food into energy, preferring to store it as fat for a rainy day! And although we might register a weight loss on the scales, we would be losing fluids and muscle, which could leave us looking gaunt and flabby. Then as soon as we returned to our normal pattern of eating we would put all the weight back on, plus more, because our metabolic rate will have fallen and therefore our body will require less food to function than before – a disaster for any slimmer!

It really upsets me when people attempt to crash diet since there really is no need. Instead, we can eat well and lose body fat by following a low-fat diet. Going on a crash diet is as much a waste of time as trying to get rich by gambling. People very rarely win!

We can speed up our metabolic rate quite easily by increasing the amount of lean muscle tissue in our bodies through regular exercise combined with a good nutritious diet, high in volume, and eaten within a regular daily meal pattern. Even if you think you have a low metabolic rate, there is a great deal that you *can* do to help boost your metabolism and start operating on a much more efficient basis – one where your body burns excess fat and utilises the food that you *do* eat as energy-burning fuel.

By the end of this four-week *Beach Body Plan*, your flame will be positively roaring! The encouraging news too is that once you have 'kick-started' your metabolism, it is much easier to maintain it. So having achieved your 'new' body, you needn't lose it again providing you don't fall back into those old bad habits that made you unfit, overweight and unhealthy in the first place.

STAGE 3

Changes For The Better

If you are going to succeed over the next four weeks, then you need to start developing some good habits. From time to time many of us make resolutions to adopt good habits such as taking the dog for a walk twice a day, giving up chocolate, or keeping the home tidier. We start off with the best of intentions then, often for no apparent reason, our determination seems to diminish and the bad habits start creeping in again. This is *so* true of diet and exercise campaigns. We start the diet with willpower as strong as iron. We wouldn't even dream of eating chips or eating between meals. Then one day we have 'just a tiny portion of chips' or 'just one biscuit' with a cup of tea . . . 'That won't hurt,' we tell ourselves, and before we know where we are we have acquired a bad habit which has to be broken if we are to succeed.

It's the same with exercise. We make a resolution to join an exercise class or take up a sport, but as soon as we miss just one game or class, it is all too easy to let other distractions prevent us from going to the next session. Once we have broken the habit of attending our weekly exercise class or game of squash it becomes much harder to get back into the routine. Physical activity should form part of our lifestyle, so we should continuously be aware of demands on our time creeping in to what should be a sacred part of our routine.

Over the next four weeks try to make some real changes to your everyday habits. Start walking up the stairs in preference to taking the lift. Park your car in the furthest, not the nearest, car-parking space to the office or the shops. Even if you have no special reason to go out during your lunch break, go for a walk rather than sitting and reading a magazine. Walk rather than drive to school to pick up the children – the extra exercise will benefit them too.

With this *Beach Body Plan* you will need to undertake some form of physical activity for approximately 30 minutes on five days out of every seven if you are to see a dramatic improvement in your body shape and a significant reduction in body fat. Plan your physical activity schedule in advance (see Stages 5 and 7 for more advice). I have left space on each day of the *Beach Body Plan* for you to write down the exercise/activity you plan to take, the time of day you have allocated and the duration. Write down 'rest day' on the two days each week when you will not be undertaking any formal exercise/activity. Transfer these dates and times to your diary and make sure you honour them.

Before deciding which activities you are going to do, consider which ones can be undertaken with other people and which should be done alone. In addition, while it is preferable to 'cross train', that is to undertake a variety of activities that use different muscle groups, you could if you wish stick to a single activity that you find convenient and that you really enjoy. Enjoyment is the key, and even if you planned to go cycling on one day but end up going swimming, it really does not matter, just as long as you do something. If you enjoy your physical activity you are much more likely to continue for the duration of the four-week plan and hopefully beyond, so that it becomes part of your regular lifestyle. Let's hope the good habits that you start now might pave the way towards habits of a lifetime.

Whatever activity you choose, it should be sufficiently energetic to make you mildly breathless and cause you to perspire gently, and it should be performed at a level of intensity that is moderate enough to allow you to sustain the activity for approximately 20 minutes, allowing additional time for warming up and cooling down.

It is a fallacy to believe that you have to work out at an exhausting level, pouring with perspiration and hardly able to speak. This is certainly not the way to achieve optimum fat burning and a level of fitness that can greatly improve the standard of your health and the quality of your life. Fitness is about being able to cope with the demands placed upon you in your everyday life and having sufficient energy in store to cope with the emergencies. It is not about being able to run a marathon or swim the channel. Remember, you're not aiming to be an elite athlete.

Imagine a scale of activity ranging from 1–10. Number 1 is sitting doing nothing, and number 10 is working out at a level that is totally exhausting, uncomfortable and almost painful. To achieve maximum fat-burning capability we should aim to work out at approximately level 5–6 on this scale.

However, not everyone is able to exercise, and the question I am often asked is 'Can I lose weight by diet alone?' The results of those who have followed my *Hip and Thigh Diet* and the other diets that I have devised over the last few years have proved beyond doubt that by following a low-fat diet you can very effectively reduce the amount of fat on your body. Many of my trial teams did no exercise whatsoever yet lost dramatic amounts of weight from the fatty areas of their body. However, this book is concerned with losing the maximum amount of body fat in a specific period of time. If you combine a low-fat diet – such as the diet in this book – with *any* form of aerobic activity (i.e. exercise that makes you breathe faster and deeper) you will burn even *more* fat. Add to this some body-toning exercises to increase your lean muscle mass, and the result is an *increase* in your metabolic rate which means you will burn more calories even when you are not exercising. It is exactly this combination that is going to change your body over the next 28 days.

STAGE 4

Going Shopping

Selective Shopping

Over the last six years food manufacturers have produced a vast variety of low-fat products. In the UK we are also fortunate in being able to enjoy the benefits of clear food labelling. This is extremely helpful to anyone on a low-fat diet as we can see at a glance what proportion of fat is contained within each item. As a general rule, you should select only foods with less than 4 per cent fat content (i.e. maximum 4 grams of fat per 100 grams of the product). I say 'as a general rule' because foods such as mustard and curry powder have a fat content higher than 4 per cent, yet the portions you are likely to consume are so minimal that these foods will do little harm. So, when making your choices consider also the actual amount you will be eating of that particular food, without getting too tied down in calculating grams of fat per portion. For instance, if the label on a tin of baked beans states a fat content of 1 per cent, then a portion of 225 grams will yield only 2.25 grams of fat, which makes it an ideal choice for the low-fat dieter.

The other exception to the 4 per cent fat rule is fatty fish such as salmon, mackerel and tuna, providing these are consumed in moderation. Since the oil found in these fatty fish is of significant nutritional value I have included them in the 28-day eating plan and recommend they be eaten once or twice a week. When making your selection, please ensure that the product you buy has been canned in brine, not oil.

When shopping, always select the best low-fat alternatives, but there is no need to opt for reduced-sugar, or reduced-salt brands of foods which are already low in fat in their regular form. In other words, regular baked beans are perfectly satisfactory for the low-fat dieter, and the benefit in choosing a 'diet' brand is too minimal to be worth considering. The key to successful shopping is to read the labels and see what options are available. Through careful selection you can dramatically reduce the intake of fat in your daily diet without losing out on flavour or depriving yourself of foods you enjoy.

Always choose the leanest cuts of meat and chicken and avoid those that have been prepared in any kind of breadcrumbs. Do not choose fish that is coated in batter, and if coated in breadcrumbs check the label for fat content. Providing the fish has not been previously deep fried, a coating of breadcrumbs is acceptable. In this context fish fingers are also permitted.

Always remove fat from chops, steaks or chicken and all skin from poultry *before* cooking. Avoid sausages unless they are home-made by your butcher using the leanest meat. Most sausages contain a high proportion of fat and, even when grilled, still retain a high level. Both salami and German sausage have an incredibly high fat content, usually around 50 per cent. Likewise, pâté should be avoided too. If in doubt, check the label.

Dairy products should be considered carefully. Hard cheeses should be avoided by all except vegetarians, who should select only low-fat brands. Non-vegetarians should choose instead cottage cheese prepared without cream. Always buy low-fat brands of yogurts and fromage frais. Avoid Greek yogurt and regular high-fat fromage frais as these contain between 8 and 10 per cent fat.

Low-fat spreads can be very misleading, particularly those which are high in polyunsaturates and low in cholesterol. Most low-fat spreads contain between 25 and 40 per cent fat (butter and margarine contain 80 per cent). However, new products are now available which contain 3 per cent fat and these are acceptable. You are unlikely to want to spread these on too thickly but they may provide good alternatives for those who find it difficult to give up butter altogether.

You may eat preserves, marmalade and honey – whatever you like within reason – with the exception of lemon curd. There is no need to buy low-sugar varieties since such products tend to lack flavour and texture, leaving the dieter feeling deprived and yearning for something better. This diet aims to be high in satisfaction and low in deprivation. Similarly, I am very relaxed about dieters having a spoonful of sugar in their tea or coffee. One teaspoonful of sugar taken four or five times a day in drinks will soon be burnt off as energy, but if taken in excess it will obviously be stored as fat. I have a theory that a lot of people who have given up sugar in the past often find it very difficult to lose their excess weight because they look for sweet alternatives from a variety of sources that are far more damaging, such as biscuits and cakes. My philosophy is that if you have a little bit of sugar at regular intervals during the day your craving for sweet things diminishes. You will be surprised if you look around you at who does and who doesn't take sugar in their tea. I bet you most of those who don't are overweight!

Sauces and dressings can be a real bonus in the kitchen, whether it be a sauce that you just pour on to your stir-fried chicken, or a dressing to bring your salad alive. There are lots of low-fat options available that are well worth considering.

Bread, potatoes, cereals, pasta and rice are allowed. Ideally, bread should be wholemeal, rice should be brown (though this does take longer to cook), and pasta should be the egg-free variety (e.g. Buitoni). All varieties of cereals are allowed but do take the time to measure the appropriate quantity to ensure that you don't eat too much. Volumes of cereals vary dramatically and whilst 2 oz (50 g) Rice Krispies would give you a substantial bowlful, 2 oz (50 g) muesli would look pretty insignificant. Choose according to your taste and capacity.

Vegetables can be eaten freely but should never be cooked with fat. Most vegetables can be dry-roasted in the oven and they benefit from being parboiled first in water with vegetable stock cube added to give them extra taste and to keep them moist.

Certain dessert foods are included in the diet and should be taken as 'treats'. Meringue baskets, fruit (tinned or fresh) and jelly are all virtually fat-free and are allowed in moderation. Likewise, wonderful substitutes such as Wall's 'Too Good To Be True' ice cream provide ideal treats. We can be imaginative but we must be restrained. Just because something is very low in fat it doesn't mean that it contains no fattening power. Calories taken in excess, no matter in what form, will turn to fat on our bodies. We want to be certain that the food we take in over the next four weeks is going to be used by our bodies and burned away as fuel, not deposited around our bodies as fat.

When you go shopping always make a list and stick to it. Only buy the foods you need, and don't be seduced by supermarket ploys aimed at tempting you to buy foods you hadn't planned on purchasing. Surplus food in the fridge all too often becomes surplus fat on your waistline or hips. Just don't buy it.

If you must buy 'forbidden' foods because the rest of the family strongly requests them, then ensure these are kept well out of sight, preferably behind a locked door. It is much easier to find the willpower to stick to a diet when temptation isn't looking you in the face.

Within the 28-day plan there is a quick and easy menu option each day which requires minimum ingredients. I find it extremely helpful to have a good selection of seasonings, sauces and dressings to hand in the store cupboard and refrigerator to produce a quick, tasty and varied selection of low-fat meals for the family. For the majority of menus included in this book, there is no need to buy oil or fat of any kind. Only vegetarians should consider using a tiny drop of oil in the preparation of their meals since they will not be obtaining essential fatty nutrients from natural sources such as meat, fish and poultry.

Regular items for the store cupboard

Arrowroot
Black pepper in a pepper mill
Brown sauce
Chilli and garlic sauce
Chilli powder

Cornflour
Curry powder
Dried low-fat milk
Garlic granules and fresh garlic
Gravy powder (not granules)
Ground ginger
Herbs and spices (any kind)
Horseradish sauce
Lemon juice
Low-fat dressings (any kind)
Marmite
Mint sauce
Mixed dried herbs
Mustard (French and English)
Pasta
Reduced-oil salad dressing
Rice
Salt
Stock cubes (beef, chicken, vegetable)
Sultanas
Sweet brown pickle
Tinned mushrooms
Tinned tomatoes
Tomato ketchup
Tomato purée
Vinegar
White wine vinegar

Regular items for the refrigerator

Diet yogurt (any low-fat, low-calorie brand)
Fresh fruit
Low-fat cottage cheese
Low-fat fromage frais

Orange juice (unsweetened)
Raw vegetables
Salad vegetables
Sparkling mineral water
Tomato juice

Cooking Utensils

Every dieter will find it helpful to have the following equipment in their kitchen to help in the preparation of meals.

Chopping board and sharp knife
Garlic press
Kitchen weighing scales
Measuring jug
Non-stick frying pan with a lid
Non-stick saucepans with lids
Spatula and spoons compatible with non-stick pans
Tablespoon and teaspoon for measuring

STAGE 5

Exercising For Maximum Effect

Formulating Your Own Plan

To maximise your fat loss and improve your body shape I have designed the Beach Body Exercise Plan. The plan requires you to be physically active for approximately 30 minutes on five days out of every seven. You will see that there are six exercise modules or categories from which to select your activities each week and, in addition, there is a programme of body-toning exercises (see pages 134–46).

Ideally, try to vary your choices so that you work different muscle groups. You can combine multiple activities within one 30-minute session and also switch from one category to another. For example, in one session you could cycle (either outdoors or on an exercise bike at home) for 20 minutes and then do ten minutes of body-toning exercises. If you wish, you can choose just one activity that you enjoy and find convenient. However, bear in mind that to achieve optimum fat-burning benefits, you need to exercise aerobically for a minimum of 20 minutes each session, and you should start timing

the activity after you have warmed up, and allow extra
time for cooling down. Working harder does not neces-
sarily mean that you will be burning more fat, the most
important factor is how long you can keep going.

Increasing Your Fat-burning Capability

Before starting any form of exercise you will need to
warm up. Whatever the activity, start off very gently, and
gradually increase the intensity over a period of three to
four minutes, until you feel your heart rate has
increased. Many people have the wrong idea of how the
body burns fat through exercise and think, for instance,
that if they eat a Mars bar they can simply run up and
down stairs 30 times and burn it off. Unfortunately, the
human body is not as simple as that.

For the body to draw on its reserves of fat and convert
them to energy through exercise, it needs to undergo
certain changes. These changes do not happen instantly.
The best analogy is to compare the body's fat-burning
process with the operation of a central heating system.
No central heating system works instantly, it takes time
to warm up. The body's fat-burning system operates in a
similar manner. By doing some gentle, controlled move-
ments such as walking or marching, or by performing
very gently the activity you have chosen, you give the
body a chance to pump more blood around the muscles.
This has the effect of warming up the muscles and
making them more effective and efficient as well as help-
ing prevent injury. Think of it this way. If you wanted to
model some plasticine, first you would 'warm it up' by
moulding it into your hand and then stretching and
moulding it into a more pliable state. In the same way,

muscles need warming up to make them more pliable and help prevent damage, and this is achieved through gentle activity followed by some preparatory stretches. Once the body's 'central heating system' is fully operational and its 'radiators' (muscles) are warm, then the body is ready to convert fat into energy that will be expended or burned away for the duration of the workout.

Of course, science is never simple, and it would be inaccurate to say that warming up prior to exercising is all you need to ensure that you burn fat when you work out. There is another element required to enable the fat-burning process to take place. The good news is that this additional element is carbohydrate, the main energy fuel used by the muscles during exercise. Our daily diet should include plenty of complex carbohydrates (foods such as bread, cereals, potatoes, pasta and rice), and we should always ensure that we eat a high-carbohydrate snack within a few hours prior to exercising (although not a large meal within an hour before). If you exercise on an empty stomach the body's fat-burning capability will decrease. This is why you may see exercise teachers who work out for hours a day, several days a week, yet who are overweight. Unless you eat regular meals, high in complex carbohydrates, the body will not effectively draw on its fat stores during your workout.

Research has also proved that drinking plenty of water prior to and during physical activity will greatly enhance your ability to continue for longer, since dehydration is one of the main causes of fatigue. Remember that tea and coffee are dehydrating, so don't drink these as a substitute for water in this instance.

Just as it is essential to warm up the body in preparation for exercise, it is equally important to gradually cool it down again. You should never stop suddenly when exercising as this could cause dizziness or fainting. Slow down gradually and then stretch out the muscles you have been using in order to prevent muscle soreness the next day.

Body Toning

In addition to aerobic activity you need to do some toning/resistance exercises (see pages 134–46) at least twice a week for the 28-day period. These can be done in addition to your five workouts, either on the same days, or you could undertake to perform one toning session on one of your rest days. However, it is important to rest completely on one day a week. These toning exercises will work your muscles in a completely different manner from the aerobic activities listed in the exercise modules. They should be performed slowly and rhythmically and repeated several times. The number of repetitions you can do will vary according to your individual strength, and only you can calculate how many you should do. You should aim to do enough of each exercise to make your muscles feel tired but not painful. For example, if you attempt twelve curl-ups but find the last two agonizing, then just do ten, have a rest and then do another ten. Try to do two sets of each exercise to gain maximum benefit. As each day goes by you will find that you can increase the number of repetitions and sets as your muscles become stronger.

Stretching

Remember, at the end of your physical activity it is important to stretch out the muscles you have been using. The main muscles to be worked in exercise modules 1, 2 and 3 (see page 129) are the large muscles of the legs. Performing the three simple leg-stretching exercises on pages 131–33 at the end of these activities should prevent any stiffness. I have also included some additional stretches at the end of the body-toning exercises (see pages 141–46).

28-day Beach Body Plan

The Diet

Each day select one breakfast, one lunch, one dinner and one 'treat' from the menus offered. Use only the menus contained in this book for the duration of the plan.

If you prefer, the dinner menu may be taken at lunchtime and the lunch menu in the evening. You may also swap any of the meals for a similar one from another day to suit your taste and convenience, providing you exchange like with like, e.g. one lunch menu for another lunch menu. Your 'treat' may be taken as an evening snack or as a dessert to accompany the dinner menu.

Unrestricted quantities of salad items and vegetables (including potatoes) may be eaten with the lunch and dinner menus. Any vegetables should be prepared and served without fat.

Do not eat between meals, but eat sufficient at mealtimes to satisfy your appetite. Fill up on extra vegetables and salad items if necessary.

Daily Nutritional Requirements

When selecting your menus, do vary your choices of food each day to ensure an adequate assortment of nutrients and a variety of tastes which prevents boredom from setting in. Each day try to incorporate the following minimum quantities:

6 oz (150 g) protein food (fish, poultry, meat, cottage cheese, baked beans).
12 oz (300 g) vegetables (including salad).
6 oz (150 g) carbohydrate (bread, cereals, potatoes, rice, pasta).
½ pint/10 fl oz (250 ml) skimmed or semi-skimmed milk.

Diet Notes

Bread: Whenever possible bread should be wholemeal. For guidance, 1 slice of regular bread from a large thin-sliced loaf weighs 1 oz (25 g). A slice from a large medium-sliced loaf weighs 1½ oz (37.5 g). The term 'light bread' means low-calorie brands such as Nimble or Slimcea.

Rice and pasta: Use brown rice whenever possible. Pasta should be the egg-free variety.

Cottage cheese: Always select low-fat brands and avoid cottage cheese mixed with cheddar and brands with cream added.

Yogurt: Diet yogurt means low-fat, low-calorie brands, any flavour. Check the nutrition panel to make sure you choose the right ones. Avoid Greek yogurt.

Fruit: 1 piece any fresh fruit means 1 apple, 1 banana, or 1 orange, or 4 oz (100 g) any fruit such as grapes, strawberries or pineapple.

Jacket potatoes: In most instances jacket potatoes are stated without a weight restriction. Unless otherwise specified, choose a weight/size to satisfy your appetite.

Sauces, dressings and condiments: All dressings should be the reduced-oil or fat-free kind unless otherwise specified in the menu plans. Gravy may be consumed in moderation if made with powder, not granules (unless a low-fat variety). The following may be consumed freely:

> Brown sauce
> Lemon juice
> Mint sauce
> Mustard (French or English)
> Oil-free sweet pickle (e.g. Branston)
> Soy sauce
> Tomato ketchup
> Vinegar
> Worcester sauce
> Yeast extract

Drinks: Tea and coffee may be drunk freely if taken black, or may be taken white provided the milk allowance is not exceeded (see page 26). You are allowed ½ pint/5 fl oz (125 ml) unsweetened orange juice. In addition, men may drink two alcoholic drinks per day and women one drink per day. One drink means a single pub measure of spirits, a glass of wine or a small glass of sherry, or ½ pint/10 fl oz (250 ml) beer or lager. Water, slimline mixers and Diet drinks may be taken freely.

The Forbidden List

Unless otherwise specified in the daily menus, the following foods are strictly forbidden whilst following the diet (some exceptions are made for vegetarians).

- Butter, margarine, Flora, Gold, Gold Lowest, Delight, Outline or any similar products.
- Cream, soured cream, whole milk, Gold Top, etc.
- Lard, oil (all kinds), dripping, suet, etc. (Vegetarians may use 1 teaspoonful of oil for cooking.)
- Milk puddings of any kind.
- Fried foods of any kind (except dry-fried).
- Fat or skin from all meat, poultry, etc.
- All cheese, except low-fat cottage cheese.
- Egg yolk (the whites may be eaten freely), except where included in a recipe or menu (although vegetarians should limit their consumption to 3 a week and non-vegetarians to 1 a week).
- All nuts except chestnuts.
- Sunflower seeds.
- Goose and all fatty meats.
- Meats products, e.g. Scotch eggs, pork pie, faggots, black pudding, haggis, liver sausage, pâté.
- All types of sausages and salami.
- All sauces containing creams or whole milk or eggs, e.g. salad dressing, mayonnaise, French dressing, parsley sauce, cheese sauce, Hollandaise sauce.
- Cakes, sweet biscuits, pastries (including savoury pastries), sponge puddings, etc.
- Chocolate, toffees, fudge, caramel, butterscotch.
- Savoury biscuits and crispbreads (except Ryvita).
- Lemon curd.
- Marzipan.

- Cocoa and cocoa products, Horlicks, except very low-fat brands.
- Crisps, including low-fat crisps.
- Cream soups.
- Avocado pears.
- Yorkshire pudding.
- Egg products, e.g. quiches, egg custard, pancakes, etc.
- Ice cream made with real cream (e.g. Cornish).

Daily Allowance

- ½ pint/10 fl oz (250 ml) skimmed or semi-skimmed milk.
- 5 fl oz (125 ml) unsweetened orange juice.
- 2 alcoholic drinks per day for men.
- 1 alcoholic drink per day for women.

The following conversion rates have been used throughout this book:

1 oz = 25 g; 1 fl oz = 25 ml; ½ pint/10 fl oz = 250 ml.

The Exercise Plan

Undertake 30 minutes of physical activity on five days out of seven (see pages 127–30). Each 30-minute session should include a minimum of 20 minutes aerobic activity. Choose activities you enjoy and plan them in advance. Remember always to warm up and cool down.

In addition you should undertake the body-toning exercises (see pages 134–46) at least twice a week.

Remember to have at least one complete rest day a week.

Day 1

Menu

Breakfast

2 oz (50 g) branded muesli with milk from allowance, no sugar.
or
1 slice (1 oz/25 g) toast topped with 8 oz (200 g) baked beans.

Lunch

1 × 2 oz (50 g) wholemeal bread roll spread with mustard or oil-free pickle and filled with
1 oz (25 g) ham or chicken plus unlimited salad.
or
1 slimmers' cup-a-soup plus 2 pieces fresh fruit and 5 oz (125 g) diet yogurt.

Dinner

1 serving Celebration Chicken (*see recipe*).
or
1 serving Spaghetti Bolognese (*see recipe*).

Treat

1 small banana chopped and mixed with 4 oz (100 g) sliced strawberries and topped with 2 teaspoons low-fat fromage frais.
or
Peel, halve and core 1 medium-sized pear and brush with lemon juice. Fill the core-cavities with 1 oz (25 g) low-fat cottage cheese and serve on a bed of shredded lettuce.

Recipes

Celebration Chicken
(Serves 4)

4 chicken portions, skinned
1 lb (400 g) new potatoes, well scrubbed
and thickly sliced
5 fl oz (125 ml) sherry
1/2 tsp paprika
5 oz (125 g) low-fat fromage frais
1 clove garlic, crushed
3 oz (75 g) low-fat cheddar cheese, grated
Salt and freshly ground black pepper

Garnish
Fresh parsley, chopped

Dry-fry the chicken for about 5 minutes until golden brown. Remove the chicken from the pan. Place the potatoes in the pan and fry until light golden brown, then remove. Return the chicken to the pan, flesh side down. Pour over the sherry. Cover with a tight-fitting lid or aluminium foil and simmer for 30 minutes.

Return the potatoes to the pan and simmer for a further 10 minutes.

Beat the fromage frais until smooth and fold in the paprika, garlic and cheese and season well. Transfer the chicken and potatoes to an ovenproof serving dish. Spread over the creamy topping and place under a hot grill until it turns golden brown. Garnish with parsley and serve with unlimited green vegetables and salad.

Spaghetti Bolognese
(Serves 4)

1 lb (400 g) lean minced beef
1 large onion, peeled and finely chopped
2 cloves garlic, crushed
1 large carrot, grated
18 oz (450 g) jar Dolmio or Ragu Bolognese Sauce
8 oz (200 g) [dry weight] egg-free spaghetti
(e.g. Buitoni)
1 beef stock cube

Dry-fry the minced beef in a non-stick frying pan until the meat has changed colour and all the fat has liquefied. Remove from the pan and drain through a sieve to separate the fat. Discard the fat and put the meat to one side. Wipe out the pan with a paper towel until all the fat has been removed.

Add the onion and cook slowly until softened and slightly brown. Return the meat to the pan, add the garlic, carrot and sauce and simmer for 10 minutes.

Meanwhile dissolve the stock cube in a pan of water and bring to the boil. Add the spaghetti and cook until just soft. Drain the spaghetti through a colander.

To serve, arrange the spaghetti on individual plates and top with the sauce.

TIP FOR THE DAY Remember to weigh and measure yourself at the same time each week on the same scales and preferably wearing the minimal amount of clothing. Record the largest measurement around your bust, the smallest measurement around your waist, the widest measurement around your hips, your widest measure-

ment (possibly around the top of your legs), the widest
measurement around the top of each thigh, and the nar-
rowest measurement around the top of each arm. Enter
the details on the Weight Loss and Inch Record Chart on
pages 158–59.

ACTIVITY

My exercise/activity for today is (fill in):

Exercise/activity	*Time*	*Duration*
....	....	....
....	....	....
....	....	....
....	....	....

Day 2

Menu

Breakfast

1 boiled or poached egg served with 1 slice (1 oz/25 g) toast.
or
1 oz (25 g) Special K eaten dry as crisps, plus 2 pieces any fresh fruit.

Lunch

4 brown Ryvitas spread with 3 oz (75 g) salmon, mackerel or tuna in brine mixed with 1 tablespoon reduced-oil salad dressing, plus lettuce, tomatoes and cucumber.
or
Jacket potato filled with grated carrot, chopped onion, sliced tomatoes, sweetcorn and chopped red and green peppers and topped with 3 tablespoons natural yogurt. Serve with unlimited salad vegetables.

Dinner

1 serving Haddock and Tomato Hotpot (*see recipe*).
or
1 serving Chicken Stir-Fry (*see recipe*).

Treat

6 oz (150 g) fresh cherries.
or
Sandwich made with 1 slice (1 oz/25 g) bread spread with Marmite, cut in half and filled with 1 oz (25 g) low-fat cottage cheese and 1 oz (25 g) sweetcorn.

Recipes

Haddock and Tomato Hotpot
(Serves 4)

1 large onion, peeled and sliced
1 clove garlic, crushed
2 × 14 oz (350 g) tins chopped tomatoes
3 tbsp tomato purée
1 large courgette, sliced
2 tsp sugar
2 tbsp lemon juice
Salt and freshly ground black pepper
1½ lb (600 g) haddock fillets, skinned and flaked
4 oz (100 g) button mushrooms
1 lb (400 g) potatoes, peeled, sliced 5 mm (¼ inch)
thick and cooked

Pre-heat the oven to 200°C/400°F/Gas Mark 6.

Gently sauté the onion in a non-stick frying pan until the onion is soft and transparent. Add the crushed garlic. Add the tomatoes, tomato purée, courgette, sugar and lemon juice and simmer for 15 minutes. Season the tomato mixture and stir in the fish and mushrooms.

ACTIVITY

My exercise/activity for today is (fill in):

Exercise/activity　　　　　*Time*　　　*Duration*

....

....

....

Transfer the mixture to an ovenproof dish and arrange the potato slices over the top. Season. Cook in the oven for 30 minutes or until the potatoes are golden brown. Serve with fresh green vegetables.

Chicken Stir-Fry
(Serves 4)

1 chicken stock cube
12 oz (300 g) [dry weight] brown rice
4 chicken breasts, skinned and cubed
1 large onion, peeled and chopped
16 oz (400 g) jar Uncle Ben's Stir Fry Sauce

Dissolve the stock cube in a pan of water and bring to the boil. Add the rice and cook until just soft.

Meanwhile, dry-fry the chicken until it changes colour. Add the onion and dry-fry until soft. Add the sauce, cover and simmer for 10 minutes.

Drain the rice through a colander and serve with the chicken.

TIP FOR THE DAY Find a skirt or pair of trousers that fits you snugly and use to monitor your progress. Choose a garment that you won't need to wear over the next month so you can use it specifically for this purpose (wearing it on a regular basis would stretch it and give you a false sense of achievement). Try on the garment every three days. This will provide you with a very effective gauge as to how much actual fat is reducing as your inches disappear.

Day 3

Menu

Breakfast

1 oz (25 g) Special K mixed with 5 oz (125 g) diet yogurt, sprinkled with 1 teaspoon sugar.
or
Banana milk shake made with 1 small banana liquidised with 5 fl oz (125 ml) milk, in addition to allowance.

Lunch

Place 8 oz (200 g) tinned tomatoes and 3 oz (75 g) tinned button mushrooms in a non-stick pan and boil vigorously until reduced to a creamy consistency. Place on top of 2 slices (2 oz/50 g) hot wholemeal toast. Season with freshly ground black pepper.
or
1 serving Chinese Apple Salad (*see recipe*).

Dinner

1 serving Paprika Pork Parcels (*see recipe*).
or
1 serving Fish Curry (*see recipe*).

Treat

1 serving Pears in Red Wine (*see recipe*).
or
Sandwich made with 1 slice (1 oz/25 g) bread cut in half and filled with 1 oz (25 g) mackerel, or tuna in brine, mixed with reduced-oil salad dressing, plus sliced tomatoes, lettuce and cucumber.

Recipes

Chinese Apple Salad
(Serves 1)

1 red apple, thinly sliced
1 green apple, thinly sliced
1 tbsp lemon juice
6 oz (150 g) fresh beansprouts
Few radishes, sliced
2 sticks celery, sliced
1 bunch spring onions, sliced
Curley lettuce to decorate

Sweet 'n' sour dressing
$1\frac{1}{2}$ tbsp lemon juice
1 level tbsp clear honey
Few drops soy sauce

In a salad bowl, mix the apples and lemon juice thoroughly, then add the beansprouts, radishes, celery and spring onions. Decorate the edge of the bowl with curly lettuce. Mix together the ingredients for the dressing and pour over the salad; toss well and serve immediately.

ACTIVITY

My exercise/activity for today is (fill in):

Exercise/activity	Time	Duration

Paprika Pork Parcels
(Serves 4)

1 tsp vegetable oil
1 lb (400 g) pork fillet, trimmed and cubed
1 tsp paprika
2 tsp dried sage
Salt and freshly ground black pepper
1 lb (400 g) potatoes, peeled and thinly sliced
1 medium onion, peeled and thinly sliced into rings
1 small red pepper, seeded and sliced
1 small green pepper, seeded and sliced
1 tsp cornflour
5 fl oz (125 ml) unsweetened orange juice

Pre-heat the oven to 200°C/400°F/Gas Mark 6.

Lightly oil 4 × 30 cm (12 inch) squares of aluminium foil. Sprinkle the pork with paprika and sage and season well. Place a quarter of the potatoes on each foil square and top with pork, onion and peppers. Season well.

Blend the cornflour with 2 tablespoons of the orange juice, then add the remaining orange juice. Mix thoroughly and divide between the four parcels.

Fold the four sides of each foil square into the centre and scrunch together to seal. Place the parcels on a baking tray and bake for 35–40 minutes until the pork and potatoes are cooked. Serve with fresh green vegetables.

TIP FOR THE DAY Have a long, low-calorie drink each day before your evening meal. I always drink one or two cans of caffeine-free Diet Coke to help fill me up so that I don't overeat when I know I am really hungry.

Fish Curry
(Serves 4)

1 chicken stock cube
12 oz (300 g) [dry weight] brown rice
1 large onion, peeled and chopped
1½ lb (600 g) cod, skinned and cubed
1 lb (400 g) jar Uncle Ben's Indian Curry Sauce
with Crispy Vegetables

Dry-fry the onion in a non-stick frying pan until soft. Add the fish and the sauce. Cover and simmer for 15 minutes.

Dissolve the stock cube in a saucepan of water and bring to the boil. Add the rice and cook until just soft.

Drain the rice through a colander and serve topped with the fish curry sauce.

Pears in Red Wine
(Serves 2)

1 glass red wine
1 oz (25 g) brown sugar
Pinch cinnamon or ground ginger
2 ripe pears, peeled but left whole
2 tsp low-fat fromage frais

Combine the wine, sugar, spice and a little water in a saucepan and bring to the boil. Add the pears and simmer for 10–15 minutes, turning the pears carefully from time to time to ensure even colouring. Serve hot or cold with the fromage frais.

Day 4

Menu

Breakfast

2 × 5 oz (125 g) diet yogurts plus 2 pieces any fresh fruit.
or
2 oz (50 g) very lean bacon (all fat removed) grilled and served with unlimited tinned tomatoes.

Lunch

Jumbo sandwich made with 4 slices light bread spread with reduced-oil salad dressing and filled with lots of salad vegetables (e.g. lettuce, cucumber, onion, cress, tomatoes, beetroot, green and red peppers), plus 1 oz (25 g) low-fat cottage cheese.
or
A large salad dressed with Oil-Free Orange and Lemon Vinaigrette Dressing (*see recipe*) served with either 3 oz (75 g) pilchards in tomato sauce, 3 oz (75 g) tuna in brine or 3 oz (75 g) salmon.

Dinner

1 serving Chicken in Creamy Apple Sauce (*see recipe*).
or
1 serving Lancashire Hotpot (*see recipe*).

Treat

6 oz (150 g) honeydew melon chopped and mixed with 2 oz (50 g) seedless grapes, topped with 1 teaspoon low-fat fromage frais.
or
1–3 oz (25–75 g) jacket potato filled with 1 oz (25 g) low-fat cottage cheese, plus salad.

Recipes

Chicken in Creamy Apple Sauce
(Serves 4)

4 chicken breasts
1 onion, finely sliced
1 clove garlic, crushed
5 fl oz (125 ml) apple sauce
5 fl oz (125 ml) chicken stock
5 fl oz (125 ml) cider
1 tsp tarragon
2 tsp cornflour, blended with a little water
Salt and freshly ground black pepper
5 oz (125 g) low-fat fromage frais

Border
3 oz (75 g) low-fat fromage frais
1½ lb (600 g) potatoes, peeled, cooked and sieved

Garnish
Fresh parsley, chopped

Pre-heat the oven to 180°C/350°F/Gas Mark 4.

Lightly dry-fry the chicken on both sides. Remove to a casserole dish. Dry-fry the onion and garlic for 2–3 minutes. Add the apple sauce, stock, cider, tarragon and blended cornflour. Stir continuously until the sauce comes to the boil. Season well. Pour the sauce over the chicken. Cover and cook in the oven for 1 hour.

When the chicken is almost ready, beat the fromage frais into the potatoes. Place in a piping bag fitted with a large star nozzle and pipe a double border of potato round a shallow serving dish. Flash under a hot grill.

Remove the chicken from the oven, stir in the remaining fromage frais and arrange within the potato border. Garnish with parsley; serve with unlimited vegetables.

Lancashire Hotpot
(Serves 4)

1½ lb (600 g) boneless neck of lamb, cubed
4 lambs' kidneys, cored and chopped
2 onions, peeled and sliced
15 fl oz (375 ml) beef stock
2 tsp cornflour, blended with 2 tbsp water
1 tsp Worcester sauce
1 tsp dried thyme
Salt and freshly ground black pepper
2 lb (900 g) potatoes, peeled and thinly sliced

Pre-heat the oven to 170°C/325°F/Gas Mark 3.

Dry-fry the lamb and kidneys briskly in a non-stick pan until the meat is well browned. Place in a shallow casserole dish.

Reduce the heat a little and dry-fry the onions until they are soft and light brown. Gradually stir in the stock, blended cornflour and water, Worcester sauce and herbs, and bring to the boil, stirring continuously. Season well and pour over the contents of the casserole. Top with a neat overlapping layer of potato slices.

Cover the casserole and bake gently for 2 hours. Uncover. Increase the heat to 220°C/425°F/Gas Mark 7 and continue to cook for a further 30–35 minutes until the potatoes are crisp and brown. Serve with unlimited vegetables.

Oil-Free Orange and Lemon Vinaigrette Dressing
(Serves 4)

4 tbsp wine vinegar
4 tbsp lemon juice
4 tbsp orange juice
Grated rind of lemon
$\frac{1}{2}$ tsp French mustard
Pinch garlic salt
Freshly ground black pepper

Place all the ingredients in a bowl and mix thoroughly. Keep in a refrigerator and use within 2 days.

TIP FOR THE DAY   Get into the habit of looking at yourself in the mirror without your clothes on. Do this first thing each morning, first standing sideways on and then full on. As the days go by notice how your tummy is getting flatter, your hips narrower and your bottom smaller. Really look for the improvement, but don't expect miracles overnight. You didn't gain all your excess weight in just three days, so don't expect to lose it that quickly.

ACTIVITY

My exercise/activity for today is (fill in):

Exercise/activity   *Time*   *Duration*

....

....

....

Day 5

Menu

Breakfast

5 oz (125 g) diet yogurt plus 3 pieces any fresh fruit.
or
2 oz (50 g) lean ham, 2 tomatoes, plus 1 × 2 oz (50 g) fresh wholemeal bread roll and 1 teaspoon oil-free pickle.

Lunch

4 brown Ryvitas spread thinly with low-fat soft cheese and served with salad.
or
12 oz (300 g) fresh fruit salad topped with 5 oz (125 g) diet yogurt.

Dinner

1 serving Lamb Cutlets in Pernod en Papillote (*see recipe*).
or
1 serving Chicken Curry (*see recipe*).

Treat

1/4 pint/5 fl oz (125 ml) jelly made up with water, served with 1 oz (25 g) Wall's 'Too Good To Be True' ice cream.
or
¾ oz (18.75 g) toast topped with 3 oz (75 g) baked beans.

Recipes

Lamb Cutlets in Pernod en Papillote
(Serves 4)

For this recipe you will need 4 squares of aluminium foil large enough to make 4 parcels.

8 lamb cutlets, lean and thinly cut
Salt and freshly ground black pepper
1 lb (400 g) new potatoes, washed and sliced
4 spring onions, finely chopped
4 tsp fresh chives, chopped
4 tsp Pernod

Pre-heat the oven to 180°C/350°F/Gas Mark 4.

Place 2 cutlets on each of the foil squares and sprinkle the cutlets with salt and pepper. Place a quarter of the sliced potatoes, spring onions and chives on each square to cover the cutlets and pour 1 tsp Pernod over each. Wrap up each parcel very securely.

Bake in the oven for 30–40 minutes and serve with unlimited vegetables.

Chicken Curry
(Serves 4)

1 chicken stock cube
12 oz (300 g) [dry weight] brown rice
4 chicken breasts, skinned and cubed
1 × 1 lb (400 g) jar Uncle Ben's Indian Curry Sauce

Dry-fry the chicken breasts until they change colour. Add the onion and dry-fry until soft. Add the sauce, cover and simmer for 10 minutes.

Dissolve the stock cube in a saucepan of water and bring to the boil. Add the rice and cook until just soft.

Drain the rice through a colander, and serve with the chicken breasts.

TIP FOR THE DAY   Really concentrate on pulling your tummy in and walking with a better posture throughout the day. By adopting good posture habits you will be surprised how much slimmer you look and how much better you feel.

ACTIVITY

My exercise/activity for today is (fill in):

Exercise/activity   *Time*   *Duration*

....

....

....

....

Day 6

Menu

Breakfast

4 brown Ryvitas spread with 1 tablespoon marmalade or preserve.
or
2 bananas plus 5 oz (125 g) diet yogurt, any flavour.

Lunch

2 slices (2 oz/50 g) wholemeal toast topped with 8 oz (200 g) baked beans and 8 oz (200 g) tinned tomatoes.
or
1 serving Summer Delight (*see recipe*).

Dinner

1 serving Duchesse Haddock Pie (*see recipe*).
or
1 serving Navarin of Beef (*see recipe*).

Treat

3 oz (75 g) Wall's 'Too Good To Be True' ice cream, any flavour.
or
Mint yogurt dip with crudités: mix 5 oz (125 g) natural yogurt with 1 teaspoon mint sauce. Chop up carrots, celery, mushrooms, peppers, onions and tomatoes into bite-size pieces and dip away to your heart's content.

Recipes

Duchesse Haddock Pie
(Serves 4)

1½ lb (600 g) potatoes, peeled and cut into
even-sized pieces
1 lb (400 g) haddock, skinned, boned and
cut into large pieces
2 oz (50 g) red lentils
1 medium onion, peeled and roughly chopped
2 large courgettes, sliced
4 oz (100 g) baby corn, topped and tailed
2 oz (50 g) frozen peas
1 tbsp fresh parsley, chopped
4 fl oz (100 ml) milk
2 tsp cornflour, mixed with 2 tbsp water
1 tbsp tomato ketchup
Salt and freshly ground black pepper

Place the potatoes in a pan of cold water, bring to the boil and then simmer for 15–20 minutes or until cooked. Drain, mash well and season.

Place the haddock and lentils in a shallow pan with 12 fl oz (300 ml) water. Bring to the boil and simmer for 7–10 minutes or until the fish is just cooked. Strain off the liquor and reserve.

Dry-fry the onion and courgettes in a non-stick frying pan until soft. Add the baby corn and cook for a further 2 minutes. Add the fish liquor then stir in the peas, parsley and milk. Season well. Simmer for 5–10 minutes or until the vegetables are just tender. Remove from the heat and gradually add the cornflour mixture. Return to the heat and bring to the boil, stirring continuously.

Place the mashed potato in a piping bag with a large star nozzle. Pipe rosettes around the edge of a shallow ovenproof dish. Make a small dip in the top of each rosette with the end of a spoon. Fill each dip with a little tomato ketchup. Grill for 4–5 minutes or until the potato has browned.

Add the fish and lentils to the vegetable mixture and cook for a further 3 minutes. Season well. Spoon the mixture into the centre of the serving dish and serve piping hot with additional vegetables or a mixed salad.

Navarin of Beef
(Serves 4)

1 lb (400 g) lean braising steak, trimmed and cubed
1 clove garlic, crushed
8 oz (200 g) button onions, peeled
1 tbsp fresh rosemary, chopped
1½ pints (750 ml) beef stock
1 lb (400 g) potatoes, peeled and cut into chunks
8 oz (200 g) carrots, cut into large strips
8 oz (200 g) turnips, cut into large chunks
½ tbsp cornflour, blended with 2 tbsp water (optional)
4 oz (100 g) frozen peas
4 oz (100 g) frozen broad beans
4 tbsp fresh parsley, chopped
Salt and freshly ground black pepper

Pre-heat the oven to 180°C/350°F/Gas Mark 4.

Heat a non-stick casserole dish and sauté the steak with the garlic and onions until the meat is browned. Add the rosemary, pour in the stock, cover and cook in the oven for 45 minutes.

Add the potatoes, carrots and turnips and cook for a further 40 minutes. Thicken if necessary with the blended cornflour. Stir in the peas, beans and parsley. Season well and cook for a further 20 minutes. Serve as a complete meal.

Summer Delight
(Serves 2)

5 oz (125 g) fruit-flavoured diet yogurt
1 pint (500 ml) jelly, made up with water
4 oz (100 g) low-fat cottage cheese
8 oz (200 g) fresh fruit of your choice
2 oz (50 g) Wall's 'Too Good To Be True' ice cream

Spoon alternate layers of yogurt, jelly, cottage cheese, fruit and ice cream into a large sundae glass. Garnish with some extra fruit and serve immediately.

TIP FOR THE DAY Remember, you can swap around any of the menus in this book so that you eat only foods that you enjoy and that fit in with your lifestyle. Doing so will ensure you stick to the diet and achieve success.

ACTIVITY

My exercise/activity for today is (fill in):

Exercise/activity	*Time*	*Duration*

Day 7

Menu

Breakfast

4 oz (100 g) tinned peaches in natural juice plus 5 oz (125 g) diet yogurt, any flavour.
or
2 Weetabix with 5 fl oz (125 ml) milk in addition to allowance, plus 2 teaspoons sugar.

Lunch

Cheesy banana sandwich: mash 1 banana with 2 oz (50 g) low-fat cottage cheese and spread it on a thin slice (1 oz/50 g) of wholemeal bread. Top with another slice of bread and cut into triangles. Serve immediately.
or
1 serving Mixed Vegetable Soup (*see recipe*) plus 1 × 2 oz (50 g) wholemeal bread roll.

Dinner

1 serving Moray Chicken (*see recipe*).
or
1 serving Chilli Con Carne (*see recipe*).

Treat

1 kiwi fruit plus 5 oz (125 g) diet yogurt.
or
A large salad tossed in reduced-oil salad dressing, served with 2 oz (50 g) low-fat cottage cheese.

Recipes

Mixed Vegetable Soup
(Serves 4)

4 oz (100 g) old but firm potatoes, peeled and grated
4 oz (100 g) carrots, peeled and grated
4 oz (100 g) onions, peeled and finely sliced
4 oz (100 g) leeks, finely sliced
1–2 sticks celery, finely sliced
2 pints (1.2 litres) chicken stock
Salt and freshly ground black pepper

Garnish
Fresh parsley or chives, chopped

Place the vegetables in a large pan with the chicken stock. Season well. Bring to the boil, cover and simmer gently for 20–30 minutes until all the vegetables are tender. If you prefer a smooth soup, purée the vegetables in a food processor or liquidiser or through a vegetable mill.

Add more stock to thin the soup if necessary. Check the seasoning, reheat and pour into a hot soup tureen.

Garnish with fresh parsley or chives and serve hot.

ACTIVITY

My exercise/activity for today is (fill in):

Exercise/activity	*Time*	*Duration*

Moray Chicken
(Serves 4)

4 chicken breasts, skinned and boned
2 medium onions, peeled and chopped
2 sticks celery, diced
2 medium carrots, thinly sliced
1 lb (400 g) potatoes, peeled and cubed
5 fl oz (125 ml) white wine
5 fl oz (125 ml) chicken stock
Salt and freshly ground black pepper
1 tsp cornflour, blended with a little water
5 oz (125 g) low-fat fromage frais

Garnish
Fresh parsley, chopped

Lightly dry-fry the chicken to seal. Add the vegetables to the pan and sauté for 5 minutes. Pour in the wine and stock. Season well. Bring to the boil, cover and simmer gently for 45 minutes. With a slotted spoon remove the chicken and vegetables to a serving dish.

Pour the blended cornflour into the pan, stirring continuously. Bring back to the boil and check seasoning. Blend the fromage frais into the sauce and pour over the chicken. Garnish with parsley and serve with fresh green vegetables.

Chilli Con Carne
(Serves 4)

1 beef stock cube
12 oz (300 g) [dry weight] brown rice
1 lb (400 g) lean minced beef
2 cloves garlic, crushed
1 large onion, peeled and chopped
1 tsp chilli powder
8 oz (200 g) tin red kidney beans, drained
16 oz (400 g) tinned chopped tomatoes

Dry-fry the meat with the garlic in a non-stick frying pan. Drain off the fat, and set the meat aside. Add the onion and dry-fry until soft. Return the meat and garlic to the pan and add the tomatoes, chilli powder and kidney beans. Cover and simmer for 10 minutes.

Meanwhile dissolve the stock cube in a saucepan of water and bring to the boil. Add the rice and cook until just soft.

Drain the rice through a colander and serve topped with the chilli mixture.

TIP FOR THE DAY When preparing mince dishes, always dry-fry the mince first in a non-stick pan. When the meat has changed colour, remove from the pan and drain through a sieve to separate the fat. Wipe out the pan with a paper towel, before returning the mince to the pan and adding the remaining ingredients.

Day 8

Menu

Breakfast

1½ oz (37.5 g) bran flakes or Fruit 'n Fibre, plus 5 fl oz (125 ml) milk in addition to allowance.
or
5 tinned prunes in natural juice, plus ½ slice (½ oz/ 12.5 g) toast spread with 1 teaspoon marmalade.

Lunch

Triple-decker sandwich made using 3 slices light bread spread with oil-free sweet pickle plus mustard, ketchup or reduced-oil salad dressing. Spread middle slice on both sides. Fill with 1 oz (25 g) turkey or chicken breast roll, or 2 oz (50 g) low-fat cottage cheese, plus lettuce, tomatoes, cucumber and sliced Spanish onion.
or
2 medium bananas and 2 kiwi fruits, sliced and served together with 5 oz (125 g) low-fat fromage frais, any flavour, or 5 oz (125 g) diet yogurt.

Dinner

1 serving Pork and Apple Surprises (*see recipe*).
or
6 oz (150 g) roast chicken plus Dry-Roast Potatoes (*see recipe*) and unlimited vegetables.

Treat

1 oz (25 g) Special K eaten dry as crisps.
or
1 chicken drumstick, no skin, plus tomatoes, lettuce and cucumber and 1 teaspoon oil-free sweet pickle.

Recipes

Pork and Apple Surprises
(Serves 4)

1½ oz (37.5 g) sage and onion stuffing mix
12 oz (300 g) potatoes, peeled and thinly sliced
1 onion, peeled and sliced
1 cooking apple, peeled and sliced
4 pork chops
1 tsp herbes de Provence
Salt and freshly ground black pepper

Garnish
Fresh parsley, chopped

Pre-heat the oven to 200°C/400°F/Gas Mark 6.
   Mix the sage and onion stuffing mix with 5 fl oz (125 ml) boiling water and leave to stand for 15 minutes.
   On four large pieces of foil, place the sliced potatoes, onion, apple and a pork chop. Top with the stuffing mix. Sprinkle with herbs and season well. Seal the parcels securely. Place on a baking tray and cook for 45–50 minutes until pork chops are tender. Garnish with parsley and serve with unlimited vegetables.

Dry-Roast Potatoes

Choose medium potatoes of even size. Peel, then blanch them by putting into cold salted water and bringing to the boil. Drain thoroughly, lightly scratch the surface of each potato with a fork, and sprinkle lightly with salt. Place in a non-stick baking tray, without fat, in a moderate oven (200°C/400°F/Gas Mark 6) for about 1–1½ hours.

TIP FOR THE DAY Is there someone else in your family you feel will also benefit from the diet? If so, let them know just how much food you are eating and how much better you feel. If you set a good example then, hopefully, they will follow suit and join you. However, we can never force anyone else to follow a diet. Each person has to make that decision for themselves.

ACTIVITY

My exercise/activity for today is (fill in):

Exercise/activity   *Time* *Duration*

....

....

....

....

Day 9

Menu

Breakfast

1/2 melon topped with 5 oz (125 g) diet yogurt, any flavour.

or

2 oz (50 g) cured chicken or turkey breast or 2 oz (50 g) smoked turkey, plus 2 tomatoes and 1 × 2 oz (50 g) wholemeal bread roll.

Lunch

4 brown Ryvitas spread with Marmite and topped with 6 oz (150 g) low-fat cottage cheese, any flavour, plus tomatoes and unlimited salad vegetables.

or

2 pieces any fresh fruit plus 2 × 5 oz (125 g) diet yogurts, any flavour.

Dinner

1 serving Tuna and Pasta à la King (*see recipe*).

or

1 chicken breast microwaved or baked with all skin removed, plus 1 serving Mediterranean Potatoes (*see recipe*) and unlimited vegetables or salad.

Treat

1 green or red pepper cored and seeded, and stuffed with 3 oz (75 g) low-fat cottage cheese.

or

1 Weetabix with 3 fl oz (75 ml) milk in addition to allowance and 1 teaspoon sugar.

Recipes

Tuna and Pasta à la King
(Serves 4)

4 oz (100 g) [dry weight] fusilli pasta, uncooked
8 oz (200 g) tin tuna in brine, drained
8 fl oz (200 ml) skimmed or semi-skimmed milk
1 × ¾ oz (18.75 g) packet of white sauce
Salt and freshly ground black pepper
4 oz (100 g) frozen broccoli, chopped

Mix the white sauce powder with the milk until it is
smooth, then combine all the ingredients in a non-stick
saucepan with 1 pint (500 ml) water and bring to the boil
stirring continuously. Once boiling, reduce the heat and
allow to simmer in a covered pan for 10 minutes.
Remove the lid and continue cooking until the mixture
becomes a creamy consistency. Serve hot with unlimited
salad.

ACTIVITY

My exercise/activity for today is (fill in):

Exercise/activity	Time	Duration

Mediterranean Potatoes
(Serves 4)

1½ lb (600 g) potatoes, peeled and cut into
even-sized pieces
1 clove garlic, crushed
1 onion, peeled and sliced
4 oz (100 g) mushrooms, sliced
½ green pepper, seeded and sliced
14 oz (350 g) tinned tomatoes
2 tsp demerara sugar
1 tsp Italian seasoning or mixed herbs
Salt and freshly ground black pepper
2 oz (50 g) fresh breadcrumbs
1 tbsp sage and onion stuffing mixture

Garnish
Fresh parsley, chopped

Simmer the potatoes in salted water until tender. Drain.

Dry-fry the garlic, onion, mushrooms and pepper for about 5 minutes until soft. Add the tomatoes, chopping them up slightly, together with the sugar and seasoning. Simmer for about 10 minutes.

Mix the breadcrumbs and stuffing together and sprinkle them on a baking tray and place in a medium oven for 4–5 minutes or until crisp and brown.

Place the potatoes in a warm dish. Pour the vegetable mixture over them and sprinkle with the crispy breadcrumb mixture. Garnish with parsley and serve.

TIP FOR THE DAY If you desperately need something to nibble between meals, peel and chop a fresh carrot and nibble away at that. It will give you plenty of munching power without sufficient calories to matter.

Day 10

Menu

Breakfast

1 oz (25 g) lean bacon (all fat removed) grilled and served with 4 oz (100 g) mushrooms cooked in vegetable stock, 3 oz (75 g) baked beans and 8 oz (200 g) tinned tomatoes or 4 fresh tomatoes grilled.

or

As much fresh fruit as you can eat at one sitting.

Lunch

2 slices (2 oz/50 g) wholemeal toast topped with 8 oz (200 g) tinned spaghetti in tomato sauce.

or

1 pack prepared salad (Marks & Spencer, Tesco, etc.), plus one of the following: 4 oz (100 g) lean ham; 4 oz (100 g) chicken (no skin); 6 oz (150 g) low-fat cottage cheese.

Dinner

1 serving Indonesian Liver (*see recipe*).

or

8 oz (200 g) fish (cod, haddock, turbot, halibut), steamed or microwaved without fat, served with unlimited vegetables and 1 serving Parsley Sauce (*see recipe*).

Treat

1 oz (25 g) All Bran with 3 fl oz (75 ml) milk in addition to allowance, plus 1 teaspoon sugar.

or

1 slice (1 oz/25 g) toast spread with 1 teaspoon marmalade, jam or honey.

Recipes

Indonesian Liver
(Serves 4)

1 lb (400 g) potatoes, peeled and diced
1 medium onion, chopped
1 clove garlic, crushed
2 tsp Schwartz Mild Authentic Curry Powder
1 lb (400 g) lambs' liver, sliced
1 tbsp plain flour
7 fl oz (175 ml) semi-skimmed milk
Salt and freshly ground black pepper

Garnish
Fresh coriander sprigs

Sauté the potatoes, onion and garlic in a non-stick pan. Add two tablespoons of water with the curry powder and continue cooking for 5 minutes.

Toss the liver in the flour and add to the saucepan. Cook until well sealed and beginning to turn crispy. Stir in the milk and 9 fl oz (225 ml) water and season well. Cover, bring to the boil and simmer for 25–30 minutes until the potatoes are tender and the mixture has thickened. Garnish with coriander sprigs and serve with salad, plus 1 pitta bread and 2 tablespoons natural yogurt per person.

TIP FOR THE DAY Have you tried on your measuring skirt/trousers recently? If not try it on today and have another assessment session in front of the mirror. Can you see the improvement?

Parsley Sauce
(Serves 4)

½ pint/10 fl oz (250 ml) skimmed milk
1 onion, peeled and sliced
6 peppercorns
1 bay leaf
Salt and freshly ground black pepper
2 tsp cornflour
Dried or fresh chopped parsley to taste

Heat all but 2 fl oz (50 ml) of the milk in a non-stick saucepan, adding the onion, peppercorns, bay leaf and seasoning. Cover the pan and simmer for 5 minutes. Turn off the heat and leave milk mixture to stand, with the lid on, for a further 30 minutes.

Mix the remaining milk with the cornflour. Strain the infused milk, add the cornflour mixture and slowly bring to the boil, stirring continuously. If it begins to thicken too quickly, remove from the heat and stir very fast to mix well. Add the chopped parsley and cook for 3–4 minutes. Serve immediately.

ACTIVITY

My exercise/activity for today is (fill in):

Exercise/activity   *Time*   *Duration*

....

....

....

....

Day 11

Menu

Breakfast

5 oz (125 g) stewed fruit (cooked without sugar) plus 5 oz (125 g) diet yogurt, any flavour.
or
Any one Variety Pack cereal, plus 2 oz (50 g) chopped fresh fruit and 4 fl oz (100 ml) milk in addition to allowance.

Lunch

2 slices light bread toasted and topped with 15 oz (375 g) baked beans.
or
1 serving Prawn and Grapefruit Cocktail (*see recipe*); plus 1 × 2 oz (50 g) wholemeal bread roll.

Dinner

1 serving Margie's Oporto Gammon (*see recipe*).
or
6 oz (150 g) chicken breast skinned and cooked in foil for 30 minutes in a medium hot oven or microwaved in a covered dish for 7 minutes on HIGH, served with boiled rice (2 oz/50 g dry weight per person) mixed with peas and sweetcorn.

Treat

1 small banana sliced into 5 oz (125 g) diet yogurt.
or
2 oz (50 g) low-fat cottage cheese mixed with 1 teaspoon strawberry jam.

Recipes

Prawn and Grapefruit Cocktail
(Serves 2)

1 fresh grapefruit
6 oz (150 g) peeled prawns
5 oz (125 g) diet grapefruit yogurt
(natural yogurt can be used if preferred)

Peel grapefruit, removing all pith. Separate into segments and place in a dish. Sprinkle the fresh prawns on to the grapefruit and dress with yogurt.

Margie's Oporto Gammon
(Serves 4)

12 oz (300 g) green, unsmoked gammon, all fat
removed, cut into strips
1 onion, peeled and chopped
1 red pepper, seeded and finely chopped
1 eating apple, with skin, cored and chopped
8 oz (200 g) tin kidney beans
4 oz (100 g) broad beans or 8 oz (200 g) tin chick peas
1–2 tsp cornflour

Sauce
3 tsp dry mustard
¼ tsp turmeric
½ tsp ground cinnamon
¼ tsp ground ginger
8 fl oz (200 ml) orange juice
1 tsp honey (optional)
3 fl oz (75 ml) white port or amontillado
Salt and freshly ground black pepper

Put the gammon, half the onion, a little pepper and 15 fl oz (375 ml) water in a heavy based pan. Bring to the boil, cover and simmer for 40 minutes or until cooked.

Mix the mustard powder, turmeric, cinnamon and ginger, add a little salt, mix in 2 fl oz (50 ml) boiling water, add orange juice, honey and port. Stir in the red pepper. Leave to stand while meat is cooking.

When meat is cooked to resistance point (rather than soft) add the rest of the onion, the apple, the kidney beans, the broad beans or chick peas and the sauce. Simmer for a further 15 minutes. Taste, adjust the seasoning, then thicken with cornflour.

Serve with jacket potatoes and salad.

TIP FOR THE DAY When cooking rice or pasta, add a stock cube to the water for extra flavour. It will also prevent the rice or pasta sticking to the pan – so you won't need to add any oil.

ACTIVITY

My exercise/activity for today is (fill in):

Exercise/activity	Time	Duration
....		
....		
....		
....		

Day 12

Menu

Breakfast

½ oz (12.5 g) bran flakes and ½ oz (12.5 g) All Bran mixed with 5 oz (125 g) diet yogurt.
or
6 oz (150 g) fruit compote (e.g. oranges, grapefruit, peaches, pineapple, pears, all in natural juice).

Lunch

Jacket potato filled with 8 oz (200 g) baked beans mixed with a little curry powder to taste.
or
Peel, halve and core 2 medium-sized pears and brush with lemon juice. Fill the core cavities with 4 oz (100 g) low-fat cottage cheese and serve on a bed of lettuce with unlimited salad vegetables.

Dinner

1 serving Chicken in Orange and Marjoram (*see recipe*).
or
1 serving Potassaka (*see recipe*).

Treat

Any one Variety Pack cereal with milk from allowance and 1 teaspoon sugar.
or
Sandwich made with 1 slice (1 oz/25 g) bread spread with reduced-oil salad dressing, cut in half and filled with assorted salad vegetables.

Recipes

Chicken in Orange and Marjoram
(Serves 4)

4 × 4 oz (100 g) chicken breasts, skinned
2 tsp dried marjoram
Salt and freshly ground black pepper
2 medium oranges
1 tsp chicken seasoning
1 lb (400 g) potatoes, peeled, cut into
matchsticks and just cooked

Garnish
Fresh parsley, chopped

Pre-heat the oven to 200°C/400°F/Gas Mark 6.

Open out the chicken breasts and sprinkle each with marjoram. Season well. Cut one orange into 4 slices and halve each slice. Divide the pieces equally between the chicken and secure the meat around the orange with cocktail sticks. Squeeze the remaining orange and pour the juice into a shallow ovenproof dish. Add the chicken and sprinkle with the seasoning. Cover and cook for 20 minutes.

Place the potatoes around the edge to make a border and cook, uncovered, for a further 15 minutes or until the potato is golden. Garnish with parsley and serve with a crisp green salad and unlimited vegetables.

Potassaka
(Serves 4)

1 lb (400 g) minced beef
1 clove garlic, crushed
1 large onion, peeled and sliced
7 oz (175 g) tinned tomatoes
1 tsp mixed herbs
1 tbsp tomato purée
Salt and freshly ground black pepper
1 lb (400 g) potatoes, peeled and thinly sliced

Sauce
½ pint/10 fl oz (250 ml) milk
2 tsp cornflour, blended with a little milk
1 oz (25 g) low-fat cheddar cheese, grated
1 tsp mustard

Pre-heat the oven to 180°C/350°F/Gas Mark 4.

Dry-fry the beef, garlic and onion for 5 minutes until browned. Add the tomatoes, mixed herbs, tomato purée and season well. Cook for 15–20 minutes.

To make the sauce, heat the milk and add the blended cornflour, and boil gently for 2 minutes. Season well. Remove from the heat and stir in the grated cheese and the mustard.

Cover the base of a greased casserole dish with over-lapping potato slices and season. Cover with a layer of the meat mixture. Repeat until all the ingredients are used, finishing with a layer of potato. Pour over the sauce and bake in the oven for 30–40 minutes until golden brown. Serve with a crisp green salad.

TIP FOR THE DAY If you are out of the house all day, it is obviously impractical to carry your milk allowance around with you. Here's a simple way to estimate how many cups of coffee or tea you are allowed. Pour ½ pint/10 fl oz (250 ml) into a jug and have another jug and a cup to hand. Pour into the cup the amount of milk you would usually have in your cup of tea or coffee, then pour it into the second jug. Continue doing this and count the number of cups of tea or coffee you could drink using that ½ pint/10 fl oz (250 ml) milk. Remember to take into account any milk you will need for cereals etc.

ACTIVITY

My exercise/activity for today is (fill in):

Exercise/activity	*Time*	*Duration*

Day 13

Menu

Breakfast

8 oz (200 g) tinned grapefruit in natural juice.
or
½ grapefruit, plus 1 slice (1½ oz/37.5 g) toast spread with 2 teaspoons marmalade.

Lunch

Jacket potato filled with 4 oz (100 g) low-fat cottage cheese mixed with 4 teaspoons tomato purée and black pepper to taste.
or
1 serving Kiwi Fruit and Ham Salad (*see recipe*).

Dinner

1 serving Hungarian Beef (*see recipe*).
or
2 rashers lean back bacon, grilled; 1 egg, dry-fried; 1 large onion, peeled, sliced and dry-fried; 3 oz (75 g) mushrooms, cooked in stock; 3 large tomatoes, grilled; 5 oz (125 g) baked beans; 4 oz (100 g) peas and ½ slice (½ oz/12.5 g) toast.

Treat

5 oz (125 g) carton low-fat diet rice pudding.
or
½ pint/10 fl oz (250 ml) skimmed milk in addition to allowance.

Recipes

Kiwi Fruit and Ham Salad
(Serves 1)

2 oz (50 g) French loaf
1 tbsp reduced-oil dressing
1 oz (25 g) lean ham

Garnish
2 kiwi fruit, peeled and sliced

Cut the loaf lengthways. Spread the dressing on the bread. Shred the ham and place on top of the bread. Garnish with the kiwi fruit.

Hungarian Beef
(Serves 4)

2 medium onions, peeled and chopped
4 tbsp tomato juice
2 tbsp paprika
1½ lb (600 g) stewing steak, cut into cubes
1 tsp caraway seeds
4 oz (100 g) potatoes, peeled and grated
2 tbsp tomato purée
½ pint (250 ml) stock
1 lb (400 g) potatoes, peeled and cubed
Salt and freshly ground black pepper

Garnish
Green pepper, seeded and sliced,
and fresh parsley, chopped

Pre-heat the oven to 180°C/350°F/Gas Mark 4.

Dry-fry the onions until brown. Add the tomato juice and stir in paprika. Add the steak, caraway seeds and grated potato. Cook for 3–5 minutes, stirring occasionally.

Add the tomato purée and stock and transfer mixture to a casserole dish. Cover and cook for about 1½ hours. Add the cubed potatoes, season and cook for a further 30 minutes. Check seasoning. Garnish with the pepper slices and parsley and serve with a large green salad.

TIP FOR THE DAY Try to be enthusiastic about the diet. Don't be a diet bore. If you are positive, others will support you, but if you're a moaner, your friends will try and tempt you off the diet.

ACTIVITY

My exercise/activity for today is (fill in):

Exercise/activity   *Time*   *Duration*

....

....

....

....

Day 14

Menu

Breakfast

1 slice (1 oz/25 g) wholemeal toast spread with 1 tea-spoon raspberry jam and topped with thin slices of one small banana. To add a luxury taste, spoon 2 teaspoons low-fat fromage frais over banana slices if desired.
or
1 whole fresh grapefruit plus 5 oz (125 g) diet yogurt, any flavour, plus 1 apple and pear.

Lunch

1 slimmers' cup-a-soup, plus 2 slices light bread spread with 2 teaspoons reduced-oil salad dressing and topped with salad and 2 oz (50 g) low-fat cottage cheese.
or
4 × 5 oz (125 g) diet yogurts, any flavour, plus 1 piece of any fresh fruit.

Dinner

1 serving Chicken with Paprika and Fennel (*see recipe*).
or
1 serving Lamb Tagine (*see recipe*).

Treat

¾ oz (18.75 g) branded muesli with milk from allowance, no sugar.
or
1 slice (1 oz/25 g) toast topped with 8 oz (200 g) tinned plum tomatoes boiled until reduced to a creamy consistency. Season well.

Recipes

Chicken with Paprika and Fennel
(Serves 4)

4 chicken joints, skinned and trimmed
1 tsp paprika
Freshly ground black pepper
1 clove garlic, crushed
4 oz (100 g) lean smoked bacon, rinded and chopped
1 small leek, sliced
1 medium head fennel, chopped
4 oz (100 g) mushrooms, quartered
1¼ lb (500 g) new potatoes, scrubbed and cut into
even-sized pieces
1 tbsp tomato purée
1 bouquet garni
1 pint (500 ml) chicken stock
4 oz (100 g) green beans, topped and tailed
4 medium tomatoes, skinned and quartered
1 tbsp cornflour, blended with a little cold water

Garnish
Fresh parsley, chopped

Pre-heat the oven to 180°C/350°F/Gas Mark 4.

Sprinkle the chicken lightly with half the paprika and
season with black pepper. Place the chicken, garlic and
bacon in a large, non-stick flameproof casserole dish.
Sauté for 5 minutes to seal the chicken. Remove from
dish and set aside.

Dry-fry the leek, fennel and mushrooms for 3–4 minutes, adding a little warm stock if necessary, and stir in
the remaining paprika, potatoes, tomato purée and bou-

quet garni. Replace the chicken in the casserole, pour over the stock and season well. Cover and cook for 40 minutes.

Remove casserole from the oven and stir in the beans, tomatoes and blended cornflour. Return to the oven and cook for a further 20 minutes. Remove the bouquet garni. Garnish with parsley and serve with crusty bread (2 oz/50 g per person) as a complete meal.

Lamb Tagine
(Serves 4)

1 lb (400 g) lamb fillet, trimmed and cubed
Salt and freshly ground black pepper
1 medium onion, peeled and sliced
1 medium head fennel, roughly chopped
12 oz (300 g) potatoes, peeled and roughly diced
½ tsp ground ginger
pinch of saffron, diffused in a little hot water
1 strip of orange peel
15 fl oz (375 ml) chicken stock
4 oz (100 g) mange tout, topped and tailed
4 oz (100 g) tinned apricot halves in natural juice,
drained and quartered
1 tbsp cornflour, blended with a little cold water
1 tbsp lemon juice

Garnish
Mint leaves

Place the lamb in a non-stick saucepan, season and gently sauté for 5 minutes stirring occasionally. Add the onion, fennel, potatoes, ginger, saffron and orange peel. Sweat for 3–4 minutes, then add the stock. Bring to the boil, then reduce to a gentle simmer and cook for 20–25 minutes.

Stir in the mange tout and apricots and cook for a further 2–3 minutes. Add the blended cornflour to the pan and stir well until thickened. Add the lemon juice and adjust the seasoning. Garnish with mint leaves and serve with grilled tomatoes, mushrooms and green vegetables.

TIP FOR THE DAY Before purchasing supermarket food products, always read the label carefully to check the fat content. If a product contains more than 4 per cent fat, leave it alone.

ACTIVITY

My exercise/activity for today is (fill in):

Exercise/activity	*Time*	*Duration*
....	....	....
....	....	....
....	....	....
....	....	....

Day 15

Menu

Breakfast

1½ oz (37.5 g) wholewheat cereal with 5 fl oz (125 ml) milk in addition to allowance and 1 teaspoon sugar.
or
8 oz (200 g) tinned tomatoes served on 1 slice (1½ oz/37.5 g) toast.

Lunch

Jacket potato served with 3 oz (75 g) low-fat cottage cheese plus unlimited salad (cottage cheese may be flavoured with chives, onion, pineapple, etc., but it must be 'low-fat').
or
1 serving Curried Chicken and Yogurt Salad (*see recipe*).

Dinner

1 serving Porc au Moutarde (*see recipe*).
or
6 oz (150 g) [uncooked weight] lean steak grilled and served with 8 oz (200 g) jacket potato plus unlimited vegetables.

Treat

6 oz (150 g) fresh pineapple.
or
1 brown Ryvita spread with 1 teaspoon raspberry jam topped with 1 oz (25 g) low-fat cottage cheese.

Recipes

Curried Chicken and Yogurt Salad
(Serves 1)

5 oz (125 g) natural yogurt
1 tsp curry powder
3 oz (75 g) chicken breast, cooked and cut into cubes
Unlimited green salad vegetables

Mix yogurt and curry powder together and stir in the chicken. Serve on a bed of fresh green salad vegetables.

Porc au Moutarde
(Serves 4)

1 lb (400 g) stewing pork, cut into strips
1 lb (400 g) potatoes, peeled and diced
4 oz (100 g) bacon, diced
1 large onion, peeled and chopped
4 oz (100 g) mushrooms, sliced
½ pint/10 fl oz (250 ml) chicken stock
½ pint/10 fl oz (250 ml) white wine
1 tbsp French mustard
2 tsp cornflour, blended with 2 tbsp water
Salt and freshly ground black pepper

Pre-heat the oven to 170°C/325°F/Gas Mark 3.
Dry-fry the pork briskly until golden brown. Transfer to a casserole dish with the potatoes. Dry-fry the bacon, onion and mushrooms in the same pan until lightly coloured, add to the casserole dish using a slotted spoon.

Stir the stock into the pan with the juices and add the wine and mustard. Stir in the blended cornflour. Season and add to the casserole dish. Cover and cook in the oven for 2 hours or until the pork is tender. Serve with fresh green vegetables.

TIP FOR THE DAY   Never eat standing up. Always sit at the table to make each meal a special occasion.

ACTIVITY

My exercise/activity for today is (fill in):

Exercise/activity	*Time*	*Duration*

Day 16

Menu

Breakfast

5 oz (125 g) diet yogurt, plus 1 slice toast spread with 2 teaspoons marmalade, jam or honey.
or
¾ oz (18.75 g) All Bran with 1 small banana, sliced, plus 4 fl oz (100 ml) milk in addition to allowance and 1 teaspoon sugar.

Lunch

2 slices (2 oz/50 g) bread spread with reduced-oil salad dressing and filled with lettuce, salad and 3 oz (75 g) prawns.
or
1 serving Fresh Vegetable Soup (*see recipe*), served with 1 slice (1 oz/25 g) toast, followed by 2 pieces any fresh fruit.

Dinner

1 serving Cheese 'n' Herb Chicken (*see recipe*).
or
1 serving Orange and Cranberry Kidneys (*see recipe*).

Treat

Banana milk shake made with 1 small banana liquidised with 5 fl oz (125 ml) milk in addition to allowance.
or
2 brown Ryvitas spread with Marmite, plus 1 apple.

Recipes

Fresh Vegetable Soup
(Serves 4)

2 large carrots, chopped
1 large potato, peeled and chopped
4 oz (100 g) cabbage, shredded
2 oz (50 g) peas
2 oz (50 g) sweetcorn (optional)
1 large onion, peeled and chopped
2 pints (1 litre) water
1 vegetable stock cube
Freshly ground black pepper

Place all the vegetables in a large pan with the water. Cover and bring to the boil. Add the stock cube and simmer for 1 hour. Add a generous sprinkling of black pepper to taste. Allow to cool, then place in a food processor or liquidiser on high speed for 15 seconds.

Store in the refrigerator until needed. Deep-freeze any surplus to requirements.

This thick soup is an easy and economical dish that is high in nutrition and low in fat.

ACTIVITY

My exercise/activity for today is (fill in):

Exercise/activity	*Time*	*Duration*

Orange and Cranberry Kidneys

(Serves 4)

1 lb (400 g) lambs' kidneys, washed,
cored and quartered
1 medium onion, peeled and roughly chopped
6 oz (150 g) mushrooms, quartered
½ pint/10 fl oz (250 ml) beef stock
5 fl oz (125 ml) unsweetened orange juice
½ oz (12.5 g) cornflour, blended with 2 tbsp water
1 tbsp fresh parsley, chopped
1 tbsp cranberry sauce
Salt and freshly ground black pepper

Border
1½ lb (600 g) potatoes, peeled and diced
½ oz (12.5 g) very low-fat spread (e.g. Promise, 3% fat)
1 tbsp fresh parsley or mint, chopped
Thin strips of zest from ½ small orange,
blanched in boiling water

Boil the diced potatoes for 10–15 minutes until soft.
Drain and keep warm.

Dry-fry the kidneys and onion for 2 minutes until the
kidneys have browned. Add the mushrooms and fry for
a further 2 minutes. Add the beef stock, orange juice and
cornflour mixture. Bring to the boil, stirring continuously, and cook for 10 minutes stirring occasionally,
allowing the sauce to thicken and reduce.

Add the parsley and cranberry sauce. Season well.
Add the low-fat spread, parsley or mint and orange zest
to the potatoes, toss until coated and use to border a
serving dish. Carefully spoon kidneys into the centre of
the dish. Serve with green vegetables.

Cheese 'n' Herb Chicken
(Serves 4)

4 × 4 oz (100 g) chicken breasts, skinned
3 oz (75 g) smoked ham, thinly sliced
2 tbsp fresh parsley, chopped
1 tsp chicken seasoning

Sauce
10 oz (250 g) potatoes, peeled, diced and cooked
½ pint/10 fl oz (250 ml) semi-skimmed milk
(in addition to allowance)
½ tsp mustard powder
1 tsp mixed herbs
Salt and freshly ground black pepper
2 oz (50 g) low-fat cheddar cheese, grated

Pre-heat the oven to 200°C/400°F/Gas Mark 6.

Flatten the chicken gently with a rolling pin. Layer the ham and parsley onto each piece of chicken, roll up and secure with cocktail sticks. Sprinkle with chicken seasoning. Place in an ovenproof dish, cover with foil and bake for 30 minutes or until tender. Remove cocktail sticks when cooked.

Liquidise the potatoes and milk together. Transfer to a saucepan and add the mustard and herbs. Season well. Heat through, stirring continuously. Remove from the heat, add the cheese and stir until melted.

Cut the chicken into slices and spoon over the cheese sauce. Serve with baby corn, courgettes and a salad.

TIP FOR THE DAY Never go shopping for food when you are hungry. You will be tempted to buy more. Always make a list – and stick to it. Don't be tempted by special offers if they're not included on the list.

Day 17

Menu

Breakfast

1½ oz (37.5 g) corn flakes, puffed rice, sugar flakes or Sultana Bran cereal with 5 fl oz (125 ml) milk in addition to allowance.

or

1 oz (25 g) very lean bacon (all fat removed) grilled and served with 4 oz (100 g) mushrooms cooked in stock, 8 oz (200 g) tinned tomatoes or 4 fresh tomatoes grilled, plus ½ slice (¾ oz/37.5 g) toast.

Lunch

Jacket Potato with Barbecue Topping (*see recipe*).

or

Large salad of lettuce, sliced tomatoes, cucumber, onion, grated carrot, etc. and 6 oz (150 g) [total weight] seafood (e.g. prawns, shrimps, lobster or crab), plus 1 serving Seafood Dressing (*see recipe*).

Dinner

1 serving Square Dance Pork (*see recipe*).

or

4 oz (100 g) liver, dry-fried with onions and 2 oz (50 g) lean bacon, chopped, served with unlimited vegetables.

Treat

1 apple and 1 pear.

or

½ serving Mixed Vegetable Soup (*see recipe, Day 7*) plus ½ slice (½ oz/12.5 g) toast.

Recipes

Square Dance Pork
(*Serves 4*)

1 large onion, peeled and chopped
1–2 cloves garlic, crushed
2 tbsp tomato purée
3 tbsp malt vinegar
$1/2$ tsp rosemary
$1/2$ tsp chilli powder
1 tsp Worcester sauce
2 tbsp honey
7 fl oz (175 ml) chicken stock
$1^1/2$ lb (600 g) lean pork, cut into thick strips

Border
$1^1/2$ lb (600 g) potatoes, peeled and diced
4 oz (100 g) natural yogurt
2 tbsp parsley, chopped
1 tbsp chives, chopped
1 tbsp mint, chopped
Salt and freshly ground black pepper

Pre-heat the oven to 200°C/400°F/Gas Mark 6.

Dry-fry the onion and garlic until beginning to brown. Stir in all the other ingredients, except the pork. Bring to the boil and simmer for 10 minutes.

Place the pork in a roasting tin and pour over the sauce. Roast uncovered for about 45 minutes, turning the pork every 15 minutes until it is nicely browned.

Place the potatoes in a saucepan, cover with cold water, bring to the boil and simmer gently for 4–5 minutes until just tender. Drain.

Gently warm the yogurt (do not boil), mix in the herbs and season. Toss the potatoes in the herb yogurt. Use to border four individual plates. Divide the pork between the plates and serve with a side salad and unlimited vegetables.

Seafood Dressing
(Serves 2)

2 tbsp tomato ketchup
1 tbsp reduced-oil salad dressing
Squeeze of lemon juice

Mix all the ingredients and use as suggested.

Jacket Potato with Barbecue Topping
(Serves 1)

1 tsp Worcester sauce
1 tbsp brown sauce
1 tbsp tomato ketchup
1 tbsp mushroom sauce
3 oz (75 g) cooked prawns or chicken
1 cooked jacket potato

Place all the sauces in a small non-stick saucepan and heat. Add the prawns or chicken and heat thoroughly. Serve on the jacket potato.

TIP FOR THE DAY Always remove any fat from meat or chicken *before* cooking. It is much easier to discard at this stage than when it is crisp and crackly.

ACTIVITY

My exercise/activity for today is (fill in):

Exercise/activity   *Time*   *Duration*

....

....

....

....

Day 18

Menu

Breakfast

1 slice (1 oz/25 g) wholemeal toast spread with Marmite and topped with 2 oz (50 g) low-fat cottage cheese.
or
¾ oz (18.75 g) All Bran plus ½ oz (12.5 g) Fruit 'n Fibre and 5 fl oz (125 ml) milk in addition to allowance.

Lunch

4 brown Ryvitas spread with 2 oz (50 g) oil-free sweet pickle and topped with either 4 slices of turkey roll or chicken roll or 3 oz (75 g) ordinary chicken or turkey breast, plus 2 tomatoes, sliced. 1 piece any fresh fruit.
or
8 oz (200 g) baked beans served cold with chopped salad of lettuce, tomatoes, onions, celery, cucumber, etc.

Dinner

Beef Teriyaki Skewers (*see recipe*).
or
6 oz (150 g) pork chop (including bone), all fat removed, served with 2 oz (50 g) apple sauce (no sugar), 2 oz (50 g) [cooked weight] sage and onion stuffing (no fat), Dry-Roast Potatoes (*see recipe, Day 8*) and unlimited vegetables.

Treat

4 oz (100 g) raspberries plus a meringue nest topped with 1 teaspoon low-fat fromage frais.
or
1 tin Heinz Weight Watchers soup, any flavour.

Recipes

Beef Teriyaki Skewers
(Serves 4)

1 lb (400 g) rump steak, beaten and
cut into 24 pieces
24 small new potatoes, scrubbed and
cooked whole
8 spring onions, topped and tailed
2 large red peppers, seeded and
cut into squares
1 tsp Schwartz Onion Pepper
1 orange, cut into 8 segments
12 oz (300 g) [dry weight] brown rice,
boiled and drained

Marinade
2 tbsp dark soy sauce
2 tbsp dry sherry
2 tsp soft brown sugar
2 tsp fresh ginger, peeled and finely grated
1 tsp Chinese five spice powder
1 clove garlic, crushed

Mix all the marinade ingredients together, add the steak
and marinate overnight in a refrigerator.

On eight skewers, alternate steak, potatoes, spring
onions and red pepper. Sprinkle the skewers with onion
pepper and cook under a hot grill for 10–15 minutes
until the steak is tender. Alternatively, barbecue until
tender.

Place an orange segment on the end of each kebab
and serve with a crisp green salad and boiled rice.

ACTIVITY

My exercise/activity for today is (fill in):

Exercise/activity	Time	Duration

TIP FOR THE DAY If you like porridge for breakfast (see Day 19), prepare it the night before (using water not milk) and leave to stand overnight. By morning it will have expanded and will therefore fill you up more.

Day 19

Menu

Breakfast

1½ oz (37.5 g) [dry weight] porridge cooked with water and served with 2 teaspoons honey, no sugar, plus 4 fl oz (100 ml) milk in addition to allowance.
or
4 dried apricots or prunes plus 5 oz (125 g) diet yogurt, any flavour.

Lunch

2 slices (2 oz/50 g) bread with 1 oz (25 g) ham, 1 tomato and oil-free sweet pickle, plus salad.
or
1 serving Fruit and Chicken Salad (*see recipe*).

Dinner

1 serving Oriental Cod with Lime and Wild Rice (*see recipe*).
or
1 serving any main course Lean Cuisine dish or similar product, served with unlimited vegetables or salad.

Treat

1 extra alcoholic drink, e.g. 1 measure of sherry, 1 glass of wine, ½ pint beer or lager, or 1 single measure of gin or whisky with a slimline mixer.
or
1 brown Ryvita spread with 2 oz (50 g) tuna in brine mixed with ½ tablespoon reduced-oil salad dressing.

Recipes

Fruit and Chicken Salad

(Serves 1)

Unlimited amounts of shredded lettuce, chopped cucumber and any other green salad.

1 apple
1 pear
1 orange
1 kiwi fruit
2 oz (50 g) cooked chicken breast, chopped

Dressing
2 tbsp natural yogurt
1 tbsp wine vinegar
1 clove garlic, crushed
Salt and freshly ground black pepper

Place the lettuce and green salad on a large dinner plate. Prepare the fruits by peeling, coring and slicing. Lay the slices in a circle on top of the salad vegetables and place the chopped chicken in the centre.

Mix together the dressing ingredients, pour over the salad and serve.

ACTIVITY

My exercise/activity for today is (fill in):

Exercise/activity	Time	Duration

Oriental Cod with Lime and Wild Rice

(Serves 2)

1 lb (400 g) cod fillet, skinned
Zest and juice of 1 lime
2 tbsp tamari or soy sauce
6 oz (150 g) [dry weight] brown rice
1 oz (25 g) wild rice
1 carrot, grated
½ courgette, grated
1 oz (25 g) mushrooms, chopped

Cut cod into 1 inch (2.5 cm) cubes and put into a dish. Mix the lime zest, juice and tamari or soy sauce. Pour over cod and leave to marinate until ready to cook.

Cook the rices together in boiling water. Drain and mix with the grated carrot, courgette and chopped mushrooms. Keep warm.

Pour the cod and the marinade into a saucepan and simmer for 10 minutes until the fish flakes.

Arrange the rice mixture on a serving dish with the cod and pour the marinade over the top. Serve immediately.

TIP FOR THE DAY Tomorrow's menu offers a slice of Sultana Cake as a treat. If you select this option you will need to soak the sultanas/dried fruit overnight (see page 96).

Day 20

Menu

Breakfast

2 slices (2 oz/50 g) wholemeal toast spread with 3 teaspoons marmalade, jam or honey.
or
Home-made muesli made with ½ oz (12.5 g) oats, ½ oz (12.5 g) sultanas or ½ banana sliced, 2 teaspoons bran, 1 eating apple, grated or chopped, plus 3 fl oz (75 ml) milk in addition to allowance or 3 oz (75 g) natural yogurt.

Lunch

Jacket Potato with Chilli Bacon (*see recipe*).
or
4–5 pieces any fresh fruit.

Dinner

1 serving Lemon Chicken Breasts on a Bed of Leeks (*see recipe*).
or
4 oz (100 g) roast beef or lamb, served with Dry-Roast Potatoes (*see recipe, Day 8*) and unlimited vegetables.

Treat

1 slice Sultana Cake (*see recipe*).
or
4 oz (100 g) any fresh fruit served with 1 oz (25 g) 'Too Good To Be True' ice cream.

Recipes

Lemon Chicken Breasts on a Bed of Leeks
(Serves 2)

1 small rasher of bacon
3 oz (75 g) onions, peeled and chopped
1 clove garlic, crushed
1 oz (25 g) celery, chopped
2 oz (50 g) mushrooms, chopped
2 tbsp lemon juice
1 tbsp soy sauce
2 oz (50 g) fresh breadcrumbs
1 tbsp thyme, chopped
1 tbsp parsley, chopped
1 egg, beaten
2 chicken breasts, skinned and boned
Fat-reduced chicken stock cube
2 tbsp sherry
1 lb (400 g) leeks, roughly chopped

Garnish
Lemon slices and parsley sprigs

In a non-stick frying pan, gently heat the bacon, onions and garlic. Add celery, mushrooms, lemon juice and soy sauce. Cook gently until vegetables are almost cooked through (if more liquid is required, add warm water). Remove from heat.

Combine the breadcrumbs and herbs in a dish with a small amount of warm water, to a dropping consistency, and then add this to the vegetable and bacon mix. Add half the beaten egg to bind (discard the rest). Cool in the refrigerator.

Pre-heat the oven to 180°C/350°F/Gas Mark 4.

Carefully slice the chicken breasts to within ½ inch (1 cm) of edge and open out like a book. Place a sheet of cling film over the chicken breasts and gently beat until they are ¼ in (5 mm) thick and roughly rectangular.

Remove the cling film and spread the chilled stuffing to within ½ inch (1 cm) of the edge of the breasts and carefully roll lengthways (like a Swiss roll), tie with thin string at 1 inch (2.5 cm) intervals, then tuck and tie the ends of the breasts under the roll. Chill whilst preparing the poaching liquid.

Make the poaching liquid by dissolving the stock cube in ½ pint/10 fl oz (250 ml) hot water, add the sherry and pour into an ovenproof dish. Quickly brown the chicken rolls in a non-stick pan and place in the hot poaching liquid.

Bake uncovered in the oven for 20–25 minutes. Meanwhile, steam and then purée the leeks. Remove the chicken from the oven and after allowing to 'settle' for a few minutes in a warm place, slice at a slight angle to reveal the stuffing. Fan and place on a bed of leeks. Serve with a slice of lemon and a sprig of parsley on each portion, with unlimited vegetables.

ACTIVITY

My exercise/activity for today is (fill in):

Exercise/activity	*Time*	*Duration*

Jacket Potato with Chilli Bacon
(Serves 1)

1 oz (25 g) lean bacon, chopped
1 small onion, peeled and chopped
4 mushrooms, chopped
2 tbsp chilli sauce
1 cooked jacket potato, halved and opened

Dry-fry the bacon, onion and mushrooms in a non-stick frying pan. When cooked, add the chilli sauce and mix well.

Pile on to the two halves of the jacket potato. Serve immediately.

Sultana Cake
(1 serving = ¹/₂ inch/1.25 cm slice)

1 lb (400 g) sultanas or dried mixed fruit
1 mug hot black tea
1 mug soft brown sugar
2 mugs self-raising flour
1 egg, beaten

Soak the sultanas or dried fruit overnight in the black tea.

The next day, pre-heat the oven to 160°C/325°F/Gas Mark 3. Mix all the ingredients (including the tea) together, then place in a 2 lb (800 g) loaf tin or round cake tin. Bake in the oven for 2 hours.

This cake can be frozen.

TIP FOR THE DAY In preparation for your holiday, start adding a little oil to your bath water to help moisturise your skin so that it is better prepared for the sun. Keeping the skin moisturised will help keep it supple. When purchasing sun tan creams or lotions always choose one with a sun protection factor to suit your skin type and try it out before you go away in case you have an allergic reaction.

Day 21

Menu

Breakfast

Chop 1 banana and stir into 5 oz (125 g) diet yogurt, any flavour. Add ½ oz (12.5 g) All Bran and mix well.
or
½ grapefruit, plus 3 brown Ryvitas spread with Marmite and topped with 2 oz (50 g) low-fat cottage cheese.

Lunch

Sandwich made with 2 slices (2 oz/50 g) wholemeal bread spread with 2 tablespoons Seafood Dressing (*see recipe, Day 17*) and filled with 2 oz (50 g) tinned salmon and cucumber.
or
1 lb (400 g) strawberries or raspberries plus 2 × 5 oz (125 g) diet yogurts.

Dinner

1 serving Egg and Vegetable Sauté (*see recipe*).
or
8 oz (200 g) white fish microwaved or steamed in skimmed milk in addition to allowance, served with unlimited vegetables, 1 serving Parsley Sauce (*see recipe, Day 10*) and 1 serving Duchesse Potatoes (*see recipe*).

Treat

3 oz (75 g) fruit sorbet (any brand).
or
1 brown Ryvita spread with Marmite and topped with 2 oz (50 g) low-fat cottage cheese.

Recipes

Egg and Vegetable Sauté
(Serves 4)

2 tsp olive oil
1 tbsp vegetable oil
4 eggs, beaten
1 medium onion, peeled and roughly chopped
1 clove garlic, chopped
1¼ lb (500 g) potatoes, peeled, coarsely grated, rinsed
and dried
1 medium red pepper
4 oz (100 g) mushrooms, halved
4 tomatoes
4 oz (100 g) baby sweetcorn, halved
4 oz (100 g) mange tout, topped and tailed
4 oz (100 g) broccoli, broken into small florets
1 tbsp tomato purée
2 tbsp tomato ketchup
3 tbsp light soy sauce
Freshly ground black pepper

Garnish
Fresh parsley, chopped

Heat the oils in a large non-stick frying pan or wok, add
the beaten eggs and cook as an omelette for 2 minutes.
Remove to a plate.

Fry the onion and garlic together in the same pan for
1 minute. Add the potato and stir-fry for 5 minutes. Add
the remaining vegetables and fry, stirring occasionally,
for a further 15–20 minutes until the potato is just
cooked.

Roughly chop the omelette and add to the vegetable mixture. Stir in the tomato purée, ketchup and soy sauce and cook for a further 5 minutes. Season well. Garnish with fresh parsley and serve with green vegetables.

Note: For this vegetarian recipe to work, a small amount of oil is permitted and has been taken into account for total fat content.

Duchesse Potatoes
(Serves 4)

2 oz (50 g) natural yogurt
Salt and freshly ground black pepper
Pinch of nutmeg
1 lb (400 g) potatoes, peeled, cooked and sieved
1 egg yolk, size 3

Garnish
Watercress

Beat the yogurt, seasoning and nutmeg into the potato. Place the mixture in a saucepan, add the egg yolk and mix well over a low heat until the mixture leaves the base of the pan clean.

Place the mixture in a piping bag fitted with a vegetable star nozzle. Pipe into rosettes onto a well-greased baking sheet. Brown under a grill or in the top of a hot oven. Garnish with watercress and serve.

TIP FOR THE DAY Remember, one deviation from the rules won't ruin the diet, but a huge binge could. So stop after the first lapse, forget about it and just continue with the diet.

ACTIVITY

My exercise/activity for today is (fill in):

Exercise/activity   *Time*   *Duration*

....

....

....

....

Day 22

Menu

Breakfast

1 slice Banana and Sultana Cake (*see recipe*).
or
½ oz (12.5 g) branded muesli and 1 oz (25 g) All Bran
with milk from allowance, plus 1 teaspoon sugar.

Lunch

1 × 2 oz (50 g) wholemeal bread roll spread with
reduced-oil salad dressing and filled with 2 oz (50 g)
low-fat cottage cheese, any flavour, plus unlimited salad
and oil-free dressing.
or
2 oz (50 g) ham or chicken plus 1 serving Coleslaw (*see
recipe*) and unlimited salad.

Dinner

1 serving Liver with Red Wine and Rosemary (*see
recipe*).
or
1 serving Gammon and Banana Salad (*see recipe*).

Treat

6 oz (150 g) watermelon chopped and mixed with 6 oz
(150 g) honeydew or Ogen melon.
or
1 brown Ryvita spread with a scraping of horseradish
sauce and topped with 1 oz (25 g) lean beef.

Recipes

Liver with Red Wine and Rosemary
(Serves 4)

1 medium onion, peeled and finely chopped
1 clove garlic, crushed
1 lb (400 g) lambs' liver, thinly sliced
½ pint/10 fl oz (250 ml) beef stock
5 fl oz (125 ml) red wine
1 tsp fresh rosemary, chopped
6 oz (150 g) carrots, cut into julienne strips
2 tsp cornflour, blended with a little water
Salt and freshly ground black pepper

Border
1½ lb (600 g) potatoes, peeled, cooked and mashed
1 tsp mixed herbs
Salt and freshly ground black pepper

Garnish
Fresh rosemary, chopped

Gently fry the onion in a non-stick pan. Add the garlic and continue cooking for approximately 2 minutes. Add the liver and cook for 2 minutes stirring continuously. Add the stock, wine, rosemary, carrots and the blended cornflour. Bring to the boil stirring all the time. Season well. Cover the pan and simmer gently for 45 minutes until liver and vegetables are tender.

Mix the potato, herbs and seasoning together in a bowl. Transfer to a piping bag fitted with a large star nozzle and pipe a border around a shallow serving dish. Flash under a hot grill to brown. Carefully spoon the liver into the centre of the dish. Garnish with rosemary and serve with green vegetables.

Gammon and Banana Salad
(Serves 4)

6 oz (150 g) iceberg lettuce, shredded
6 oz (150 g) lean gammon, grilled and chopped
7 oz (175 g) tinned pineapple chunks in
natural juice, drained
10 oz (250 g) small new potatoes, scrubbed,
halved and cooked
1 medium banana, sliced
Salt and freshly ground black pepper

Dressing
5 oz (125 g) natural yogurt
1 tbsp fresh chives, chopped

Place the lettuce on a large serving plate. Put the rest of
the salad ingredients into a bowl, season and toss well.

Mix together the yogurt and chives and pour over the
salad. Toss gently to coat all the ingredients. Place on the
lettuce and serve.

Coleslaw
(Serves 4)

2 large carrots, peeled and grated
8 oz (200 g) white cabbage, grated
1 Spanish onion, peeled and finely chopped
4 fl oz (100 ml) reduced-oil dressing

Mix the vegetables together in a bowl with the reduced-
oil dressing. Serve immediately or keep chilled and eat
within 2 days.

Banana and Sultana Cake

(1 serving = ¹/₂ inch/1.25 cm slice)

1 lb 3 oz (475 g) ripe bananas (5 large), peeled
2 eggs, beaten
4 oz (100 g) sultanas
6 oz (150 g) brown sugar
8 oz (200 g) self-raising flour

Pre-heat the oven to 180°C/350°F/Gas Mark 4

Mash the bananas; add the eggs, sugar and sultanas and then mix in the flour. Place in a lined 2 lb (800 g) loaf tin or cake tin. Bake in the oven for 1¹/₄ hours or until a skewer, inserted into the centre of the cake, comes out clean. Store in an airtight tin for 24 hours before serving.

This is an economical recipe as very ripe bananas can often be purchased cheaply. Suitable for freezing.

ACTIVITY

My exercise/activity for today is (fill in):

Exercise/activity   *Time*   *Duration*

....

....

....

....

TIP FOR THE DAY Fluid levels in the body vary. Don't be disheartened if the scales sometimes seem to stick. Instead, use your tape measure or measuring skirt/ trousers as a more accurate guide.

Day 23

Menu

Breakfast

4 oz (100 g) strawberries, plus 4 oz (100 g) melon, chopped, and topped with 5 oz (125 g) diet yogurt.
or
1 slice light bread toasted, topped with 4 oz (100 g) baked beans mixed with 1 oz (25 g) lean ham, chopped, plus 1 tomato.

Lunch

3 brown Ryvitas spread with 2 oz (50 g) pilchards in tomato sauce, topped with sliced tomato.
or
Boil 8 oz (200 g) tinned chopped tomatoes until reduced to a thick and creamy consistency. Grill 2 fish fingers until thoroughly cooked, and mash them. Spread the tomato sauce on 1 slice (1 oz/25 g) wholemeal toast and top with the mashed fish fingers.

Dinner

1 serving Lamb and Mint Sauté (*see recipe*).
or
1 serving Cottage Cheese and Prawn Salad (*see recipe*).

Treat

1 serving Hot Cherries (*see recipe*).
or
1 serving Argyle Soup (*see recipe*).

Recipes

Lamb and Mint Sauté

(Serves 4)

1 lb (400 g) lamb fillet, trimmed and thinly sliced
1 clove garlic, crushed
Grated rind and juice of 1 medium lemon
10 oz (250 g) potatoes, peeled, diced and cooked
6 spring onions, chopped
4 oz (100 g) cucumber, diced
3 tomatoes, skinned and quartered
2 tsp cornflour, blended with 2 tbsp water
Salt and freshly ground black pepper
2 tsp mint sauce

Garnish
Mint leaves

Sauté the lamb gently in a non-stick saucepan with the garlic and lemon rind. Remove from the pan. Add the potatoes, onions and cucumber and sauté for 2–3 minutes. Return lamb to the pan with the tomatoes, lemon juice and ½ pint/10 fl oz (250 ml) water and the blended cornflour. Season well.

Bring to the boil, stirring continuously, then cover and simmer for 15 minutes, then stir in the mint sauce. Garnish with mint leaves and serve as a complete meal.

TIP FOR THE DAY When preparing a dessert, always serve it in a pretty dish. Food beautifully presented always tastes better and leaves us with no feeling of deprivation.

Cottage Cheese and Prawn Salad
(Serves 4)

6 oz (150 g) low-fat cottage cheese
6 oz (150 g) prawns, peeled
1 lb (400 g) new potatoes, scrubbed, quartered,
cooked and cooled
1/4 red cabbage, finely shredded
1/4 cucumber, diced
Salt and freshly ground black pepper
4 tbsp low-fat cocktail dressing (e.g. Kraft)
1/2 tsp paprika

Garnish
Lemon quarters and 3 whole prawns (optional)

Mix the cheese, prawns and vegetables together in a
large bowl. Season well. Place in a serving dish, spoon
over the dressing and sprinkle with paprika.

Garnish with the lemon quarters and whole prawns
(if desired) and serve on a bed of cucumber with brown
Ryvitas (2 per person).

Hot Cherries
(Serves 1)

3 oz (75 g) tinned black cherries
1/2 tsp arrowroot
1 oz (25 g) Wall's 'Too Good To Be True' ice cream

Strain cherries, reserving juice. Heat juice in a pan and
thicken with enough slaked arrowroot (approximately
1/2 teaspoon mixed with water) to make a syrup. Pour
over ice cream.

Serve with the cherries immediately.

Argyle Soup
(Serves 4)

2 large carrots, sliced
2 large onions, peeled and roughly chopped
4 sticks celery, chopped
1 lb (400 g) potatoes, peeled and quartered
2 cloves garlic, crushed
2 pints (1.2 litres) chicken stock
Salt and freshly ground black pepper

Place the ingredients in a saucepan and bring to the boil. Simmer, covered, for 45 minutes or until the vegetables are cooked. Sieve or liquidise the soup, check the seasoning and reheat. Serve hot.

ACTIVITY

My exercise/activity for today is (fill in):

Exercise/activity   *Time* *Duration*

....

....

....

....

Day 24

Menu

Breakfast

6 oz (150 g) fresh fruit salad topped with 5 oz (125 g) diet yogurt.

or

1 oz (25 g) lean back bacon, grilled and served with 1 slice (1 oz/25 g) wholemeal toast topped with 4 oz (100 g) baked beans.

Lunch

Jacket potato served with sweetcorn, chopped salad and reduced-oil salad dressing.

or

1 serving Stuffed Peppers (*see recipe*).

Dinner

1 serving Pork Ragoût (*see recipe*).

or

6 oz (150 g) roast chicken served with peas, sweetcorn and 1 serving Coronation Potatoes (*see recipe*).

Treat

5 fl oz (125 ml) jelly, made up with water, served with 1 small banana, chopped, plus 1 teaspoon low-fat fromage frais.

or

1 brown Ryvita spread with a scraping of horseradish sauce and topped with 1 oz (25 g) mashed-up mackerel.

Recipes

Stuffed Peppers
(Serves 4)

2 red peppers
2 green peppers
6 oz (150 g) low-fat cottage cheese
8 oz (200 g) new potatoes, well scrubbed,
diced and cooked
1 tbsp chives, chopped
1 tbsp parsley, chopped
Salt and freshly ground black pepper

To serve
Fresh watercress

Cut away a thin slice from the stem end of each pepper. Remove core and seeds and wash.

Blend together all the other ingredients and season well. Stuff the mixture into the peppers, packing firmly. Chill for 30 minutes. Cut the peppers into quarters and serve on a bed of watercress, with a mixed salad.

ACTIVITY

My exercise/activity for today is (fill in):

Exercise/activity	Time	Duration

Pork Ragoût
(Serves 4)

1 clove garlic, crushed
8 oz (200 g) button onions, peeled
1 lb (400 g) pork fillet, trimmed and cubed
4 oz (100 g) button mushrooms
6 oz (150 g) courgettes, cut in julienne strips
1 medium green pepper, seeded and cut into strips
14 oz (350 g) tinned chopped tomatoes
5 fl oz (125 ml) beef stock
2 tsp dried basil
Salt and freshly ground black pepper

Garnish
Fresh parsley, chopped

Dry-fry the garlic and onions for 1 minute. Add the pork and continue cooking until slightly browned. Add the remaining ingredients and season well.

Bring to the boil and simmer covered for 40–45 minutes until meat is cooked and vegetables tender. Remove lid 5 minutes before the end of cooking if necessary to allow sauce to reduce and thicken slightly. Garnish with parsley and serve with fresh green vegetables.

TIP FOR THE DAY Experiment by mixing together different flavoured low-calorie drinks. These are ideal to help fill you up more quickly at mealtimes.

Coronation Potatoes

(Serves 4)

1½ lb (600 g) potatoes, peeled and cut
into large chunks
1 clove garlic, crushed
1 small onion, peeled and finely chopped
1 tbsp Schwartz Mild Authentic Curry Powder
1 tbsp tomato purée
1 tbsp mango chutney
4 oz (100 g) tinned apricots in natural juice,
drained and chopped
5 oz (125 g) natural yogurt
Salt and freshly ground black pepper

Place the potatoes in a saucepan and just cover with cold water. Bring to the boil and simmer for 15–20 minutes until just cooked. Drain.

Dry-fry the garlic, onion and curry powder in a non-stick pan. Sauté for 3–4 minutes until the onion is transparent. Add the tomato purée and sauté for a further minute. Mix in the mango chutney and apricots and cook gently for a further 2–3 minutes. Remove from the heat and liquidise until smooth. Stir in the yogurt and season.

Pour the curry sauce over the hot potatoes.

Day 25

Menu

Breakfast

1 slice (1 oz/25 g) wholemeal toast topped with 8 oz
(200 g) tinned tomatoes, boiled and reduced to a creamy
consistency, plus 4 oz (100 g) baked beans.
or
1 large slice fresh pineapple plus 4 oz (100 g) strawberries, topped with 5 oz (125 g) diet yogurt.

Lunch

1 slimmers' cup-a-soup. 2 brown Ryvitas spread with
Marmite and topped with 4 oz (100 g) low-fat cottage
cheese, plus salad. 5 oz (125 g) diet yogurt.
or
4 oz (100 g) red kidney beans, 4 oz (100 g) sweetcorn,
plus chopped cucumber, tomatoes and onions all tossed
in a dressing made with 1 teaspoon mint sauce mixed
with 2 tablespoons natural yogurt. Serve with other
salad vegetables.

Dinner

1 serving Chilli Prawn Jackets (*see recipe*).
or
4 oz (100 g) gammon steak, grilled, garnished with 1
slice pineapple and served with unlimited vegetables.

Treat

1 large banana.
or
Half a 16 oz (400 g) tin any branded soup (non-cream
variety).

Recipes

Chilli Prawn Jackets
(Serves 4)

4 × 8 oz (200 g) potatoes, well scrubbed and pricked
1 onion, peeled and finely sliced
2 cloves garlic, crushed
2 fresh tomatoes, sliced
6 oz (150 g) courgettes, sliced
2 tsp chilli sauce
7 oz (175 g) tinned chopped tomatoes
Freshly ground black pepper
14 oz (350 g) prawns, peeled

Pre-heat the oven to 220°C/425°F/Gas Mark 7.

Place the potatoes in the oven and bake for 1–1½ hours or until soft.

Dry-fry the onion for 1 minute. Add the garlic. Add the sliced tomatoes and courgettes and fry for a further 2 minutes. Add the chilli sauce and chopped tomatoes and boil for 5 minutes. Season well. Stir in the prawns and heat through for 2 minutes.

Slit the top of the baked potatoes, open out carefully and place the filling in the centre. Serve with a large green salad.

TIP FOR THE DAY Always buy good quality fresh fruit and vegetables. These are much more appetising than bruised or old ones and their nutritional content will be higher.

ACTIVITY

My exercise/activity for today is (fill in):

Exercise/activity   *Time*   *Duration*

....

....

....

....

Day 26

Menu

Breakfast

3 green figs plus 3 oz (75 g) diet yogurt.
or
½ pint/10 fl oz (250 ml) milk in addition to allowance, plus 1 piece any fresh fruit.

Lunch

Jacket potato served with either 1 oz (25 g) roast beef, pork or ham (all fat removed) or 2 oz (50 g) chicken (no skin), plus oil-free sweet pickle and unlimited salad.
or
1 serving Smoked Duck and Kiwi Salad (*see recipe*).

Dinner

1 serving Cassoulet (*see recipe*).
or
5 fish fingers grilled or dry-fried without fat, served with unlimited vegetables and tomato ketchup.

Treat

1 oz (25 g) Wall's 'Too Good To Be True' ice cream plus 5 oz (125 g) diet yogurt.
or
1 brown Ryvita spread with prawn cocktail dressing (*see Tip for the Day*) and topped with 2 oz (50 g) prawns.

Recipes

Smoked Duck and Kiwi Salad
(Serves 4)

1 cucumber, sliced
Lettuce or other green salad
3 kiwi fruits, peeled and sliced
1–2 smoked duck breasts, thinly sliced
Raspberry vinegar to taste
Salt and freshly ground black pepper
Parsley

Wash the salad and cut into large shreds. Spread over a serving dish. Place a layer of kiwi fruit over the salad. Arrange thin slices of duck over the green fruits. Sprinkle with raspberry vinegar, season and decorate with parsley.

This dish may be made an hour or so in advance and kept in the refrigerator. It may also be made with smoked salmon, but use lemon juice with salmon in place of raspberry vinegar.

ACTIVITY

My exercise/activity for today is (fill in):

Exercise/activity	*Time*	*Duration*

Cassoulet
(Serves 4)

14 oz (350 g) tinned white haricot beans, drained
1 large onion, peeled and roughly chopped
1 lb (400 g) potatoes, peeled and cut
into even-sized pieces
1¼ lb (500 g) lean pork,
cut into 1 inch (2.5 cm) cubes
14 oz (350 g) tinned chopped tomatoes
Salt and freshly ground black pepper
1 tsp mustard powder
5 fl oz (125 ml) beef stock

Pre-heat the oven to 180°C/350°F/Gas Mark 4.

Mix together the beans, onion, potatoes, pork and tomatoes in a large casserole dish. Season well. Dissolve the mustard in the stock and pour over the casserole. Cover and cook for 1½–2 hours until the pork is tender. Serve with unlimited fresh green vegetables.

TIP FOR THE DAY A quick and easy way to make a low-fat prawn cocktail dressing is to mix 1 tablespoon reduced-oil salad dressing with 2 tablespoons tomato ketchup, plus a squeeze of lemon juice.

Day 27

Menu

Breakfast

8 oz (200 g) smoked haddock steamed in skimmed milk in addition to allowance.
or
1 wedge of melon topped with 3 oz (75 g) grapes and served with 2 oz (50 g) diet yogurt.

Lunch

4 brown Ryvitas spread with 4 oz (100 g) low-fat cottage cheese and topped with 3 oz (75 g) prawns.
or
1 serving Baked Stuffed Apple (*see recipe*).

Dinner

1 serving Herby Fish Salad (*see recipe*).
or
1 serving Vegetable Bake (*see recipe*).

Treat

1 slice Banana and Sultana Cake (*see recipe, Day 22*).
or
1 brown Ryvita or ½ slice (½ oz/12.5 g) toast, spread with 2 teaspoons marmalade.

Recipes

Herby Fish Salad
(Serves 4)

14 oz (350 g) white fish, skinned
10 oz (250 g) new potatoes, well scrubbed,
sliced, cooked and cooled
7 oz (175 g) tinned red kidney beans, drained
7 oz (175 g) tinned sweetcorn, drained
1 medium green pepper, seeded and diced
Freshly ground black pepper

Dressing
1 tbsp lemon juice
2 tsp dried tarragon or dill
1 tbsp wine vinegar

Garnish
Fresh parsley, chopped

Poach the fish in a covered pan with a little water for approximately 8 minutes. Remove any bones and flake roughly. Cool.

Place the potatoes, kidney beans, sweetcorn and diced pepper in a bowl, add the fish and season well.

Put the dressing ingredients into a jar and shake it vigorously. Pour over the salad and toss gently until well coated. Garnish with parsley and serve.

TIP FOR THE DAY Vegetables taste even better if cooked in water with a vegetable stock cube. Save the vegetable water and season well – it can be used as an instant soup later.

Vegetable Bake
(Serves 1)

Selection of vegetables (e.g. carrots, parsnips,
peas, cabbage, leeks, onions), cooked
1 tsp mixed herbs
3 tbsp packet stuffing mix
4 oz (100 g) mushrooms
6 oz (150 g) potato, cooked
2 oz (50 g) fresh breadcrumbs,
preferably wholemeal
½ pint/10 fl oz (250 ml) vegetable stock

Pre-heat the oven to 180°C/350°F/Gas Mark 4.

Chop the vegetables and place in layers in a large
ovenproof dish. Sprinkle the mixed herbs and stuffing
mix between layers. Slice the mushrooms and place over
the other vegetables. Then, slice the pre-cooked potato,
carefully lay across the top of the dish and sprinkle with
the breadcrumbs. Carefully pour over the vegetable
stock to moisten the contents of the dish.

Bake for 20 minutes until piping hot. Alternatively,
reheat in a microwave on MEDIUM for 7 minutes and
place under a hot grill for 5 minutes to crisp the top.

Baked Stuffed Apple
(Serves 1)

1 large cooking apple
1 oz (25 g) dried fruit
1 tsp honey
5 oz (125 g) diet yogurt

Pre-heat the oven to 200°C/400°F/Gas Mark 6.

Remove the core from the apple but leave the apple intact. Score with a sharp knife around the 'waist' of the apple, cutting through only the skin.

Mix together the dried fruit and the honey and pile into the centre of the apple where the core has been removed.

Place in an ovenproof dish and bake in the oven for about 30 minutes, or until cooked. Serve with the yogurt poured over the top.

ACTIVITY

My exercise/activity for today is (fill in):

Exercise/activity   *Time*   *Duration*

....

....

....

....

Day 28

Menu

Breakfast

1 serving Banana and Orange Cocktail (*see recipe*).
or
3 oz (75 g) fresh fruit salad mixed with 10 oz (250 g) diet yogurt, any flavour. This makes a delicious home-made fruit yogurt.

Lunch

3 slices light bread or 4 brown Ryvitas, spread with Marmite and 3 oz (75 g) low-fat cottage cheese, plus unlimited salad.
or
1 chicken leg (no skin) served with unlimited chopped salad vegetables (e.g. lettuce, tomatoes, onions, celery, cucumber) and a very low-fat or fat-free salad dressing.

Dinner

1 serving Fish and Sesame Sticks (*see recipe*).
or
6 oz (150 g) gammon steak, baked or grilled, plus 1 serving Coronation Potatoes (*see recipe, Day 24*) and unlimited salad.

Treat

4 oz (100 g) strawberries plus 5 oz (125 g) diet yogurt.
or
1 slimmer's cup-a-soup plus 1 brown Ryvita.

Recipes

Banana and Orange Cocktail
(Serves 1)

1 banana, peeled
5 fl oz (125 ml) pure orange juice

Break the banana into small pieces and place in a food processor or blender. Whizz until smooth, then add the orange juice. Blend well. Serve in a tall glass with ice and a twist of orange.

Fish and Sesame Sticks
(Serves 4)

1 lb (400 g) white fish, skinned and cut into 24 cubes
24 small new potatoes, well scrubbed and
cooked whole
4 medium tomatoes, quartered
4 oz (100 g) cucumber, cut into large dice
1 tsp barbecue seasoning
1 tbsp sesame seeds

Marinade
3 tbsp barbecue relish (any brand)
1 grated zest of a medium orange
1 tbsp dried tarragon

Mix the marinade ingredients together, add the fish and leave to marinate overnight in a refrigerator.

On eight skewers, alternate the fish, new potatoes, tomato and cucumber. Sprinkle with barbecue seasoning and sesame seeds and cook under a hot grill for 10 minutes or until the fish is tender. Alternatively, barbecue until tender. Serve with a mixed salad.

TIP FOR THE DAY Really enjoy feeling slimmer and fitter today. Make a special effort to keep busy so you don't even think about cheating.

ACTIVITY

My exercise/activity for today is (fill in):

Exercise/activity	*Time*	*Duration*

Beach Body Exercise Plan

Select from any category. You can choose to follow either just one activity for the duration of the plan or undertake a number of different activities in order to achieve maximum benefit. Remember the aim is to keep active at a moderately energetic level for 20 minutes per session, five days per week, and you should allow additional time for warming up and cooling down. At least two days a week, perform the body-toning exercises on pages 134–46, but always ensure you have one day of complete rest.

During the first three days of this exercise plan, it is important that you start gently and perform the activity or activities at a very low level, otherwise muscle soreness may ensue, and this could deter you from continuing and damage your prospects of achieving a new, leaner body over the next month. Your body is the best gauge as to how hard you should work, but the experience should be a pleasurable one.

Take into account how much physical activity you have undertaken recently. Don't go and play a game of squash if you haven't played any sport or taken part in any energetic physical activity for some years. You might overdo it and seriously hurt yourself. Start by going for a brisk walk, adding perhaps a few occasional jogging steps. However, don't get carried away by the feeling of euphoria and wellbeing that taking the first steps to fitness can bring. Many an over-enthusiastic first run has resulted in a very painful hamstring and a certificate of retirement from physical activity for life. Please don't let this happen to you. If you take it gently and prepare your body sensibly, you will be amazed at how fit you can become. Perhaps the best news of all is that your fitness level will improve quickly. In no time at all you will see quite a difference in how much further you can walk, run, cycle or swim and how much better you feel than when you first started.

When selecting your activities, do take into account the actual amount of time in which you will be physically active. For example, some team games such as rounders involve periods of inactivity. Also, bear in mind that squash is not the best form of fat-burning activity, since although it will increase your level of fitness, the intensity is quite high. So if you choose squash try and combine this with additional activities.

If you have any medical condition which gives you cause for concern, it is always wise to check with your doctor before commencing any form of exercise. Most doctors will be delighted that you are taking steps to increase your general health, but if in doubt check it out.

The Beach Body Exercise Modules

Module 1: Out and About

Brisk walking
Combination of walking and jogging
Cycling
Swimming

Module 2: Slim Gym

Exercise bike
Rowing machine
Ski-machine
Stair climber
Trampoline

Module 3: Time to Play

Badminton
Basketball
Cricket
Football
Hockey
Raquet ball
Rounders
Squash
Tennis
Volley ball

Module 4: Video Workout

Work out to an exercise video for 30–40 minutes.
Recommended fat-burners are my:
Whole Body Programme 2 (BBC)
Whole Body Programme 3 (BBC)
New You Plan (VCI)

Module 5: Work out with Others

Attend your local Diet and Fitness Club (*see page 160 for details*), or your local aerobics or step classes.

Module 6: Dance the Night Away

Ballet
Ballroom
Disco
Modern
Tap

Leg Stretches

After following any of the activities from Modules 1, 2 and 3, perform the following stretches on completion of your workout.

Hamstring Stretch

- Your front leg is straight, toes raised. Your back leg is bent, heel on floor.
- Keep your weight on the back leg and hold for 8–10 seconds.
- Repeat with the other leg.

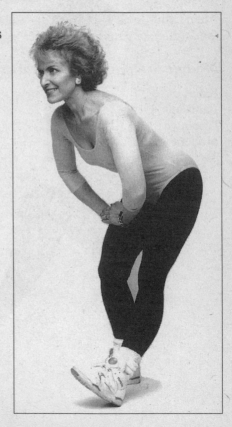

Calf Stretch

- Your back leg is straight, your front leg is bent, with both heels on the floor.
- Keep your weight on the front leg and hold for 8–10 seconds.
- Repeat with the other leg.

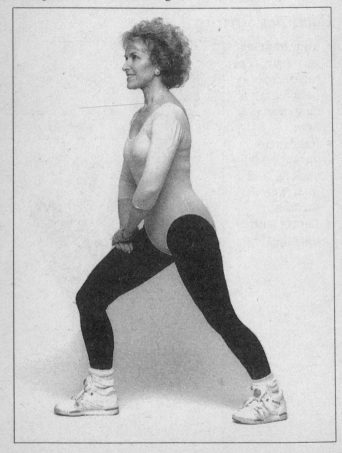

Front Thigh Stretch

- Stand on one leg, using a chair for support if necessary.
- Keeping your hips square, ease the foot of the bent leg towards your bottom and hold for 8–10 seconds.
- Repeat with the other leg.

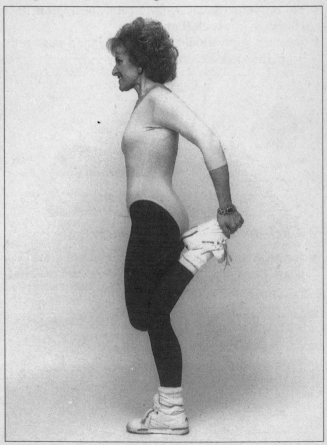

Beach Body Toning

Repeat the following exercises as many times as is comfortable.

1 Upper Back Strengthener

- Lie on your tummy with forearms resting on floor, elbows in line with shoulders.
- Squeeze your shoulder blades together, raising the arms, then release, and repeat.

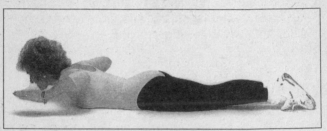

2 Curl-ups For a Flatter Tummy

- Lie on your back with knees bent, hands crossed on chest. Press your tummy into the floor and raise head

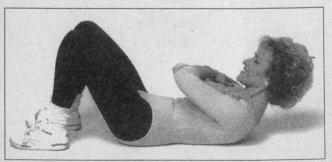

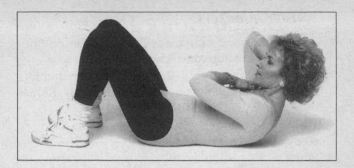

and shoulders, keeping your chin off your chest. If necessary, support your neck with one hand as shown above. Slowly lower, and repeat.

3 *Spine Strengthener*

- Lie face down with forearms and elbows resting on floor.
- Slowly raise head and shoulders off floor, and then gradually lower, using the muscles in your back, not in your arms.
- Repeat.

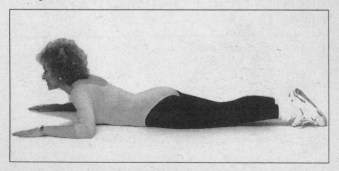

4 *Waist Minimiser*

- Lie on your back with knees bent, feet flat on floor and arms resting by your sides.
- Pressing your tummy into the floor, raise one shoulder and at the same time reach across the body. Slowly lower, and repeat to the other side.
- Repeat.

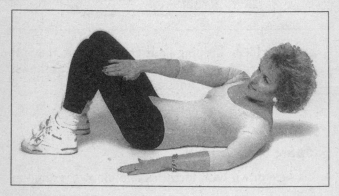

5 *Bottom Toner*

- Lie face down, head resting on your arms.
- Raise and lower alternate legs, keeping the hips on the floor and squeezing your buttocks together as you raise.

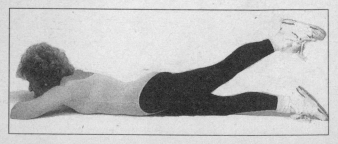

6 *Front Thigh Firmer*

- Support yourself on your elbows and bend your knees. Pull your tummy in to support your back.
- Pull one knee into your chest, then extend it out and upwards. Slowly release, and repeat with the other leg.
- Repeat.

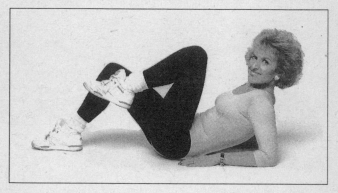

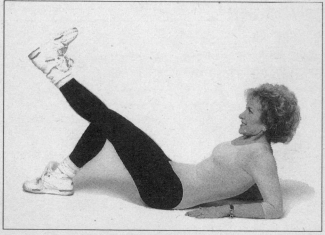

7 *Hamstring Strengthener*

- Lie face down and cross your ankles.
- Applying gentle pressure with the uppermost leg, bend and push upwards with the other leg. Slowly lower, and repeat.
- Change legs, and repeat.

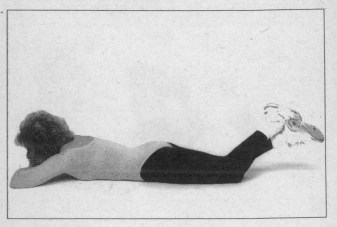

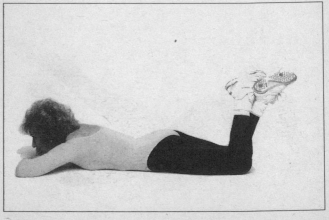

8 *Outer Thigh Toner*

- Lie on your side with hips square and lower leg bent.
- Take the top knee across to touch the floor in front, level with your hips, then push the leg out and upwards aiming the heel towards the ceiling. Release, and repeat.
- Change sides and repeat with the other leg.

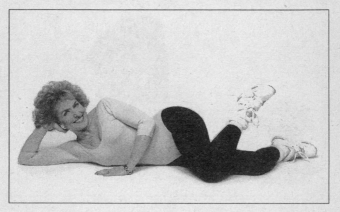

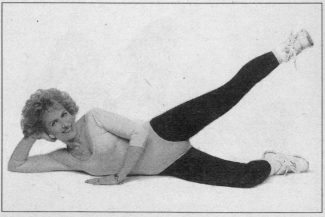

9 *Inner Thigh Firmer*

- Lie on your back with knees bent and legs raised. The knees should be directly over your hips and your lower back on the floor.
- Open the legs and close them. Repeat.

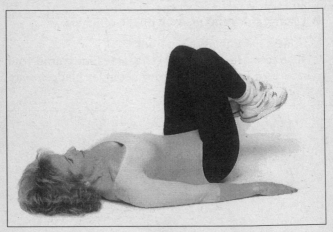

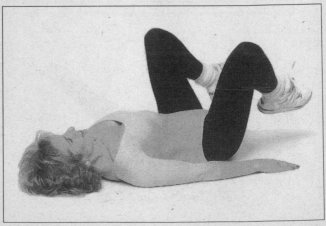

Stretches

It is important to stretch out the muscles that have been worked. The following stretches should be held for approximately 8–10 seconds. Perform each stretch once only.

1. *Upper Back Stretch*

- Sit with hands clasped in front.
- Reach arms forward and at the same time round your back as if trying to pull your shoulder blades apart. Hold for 8–10 seconds.

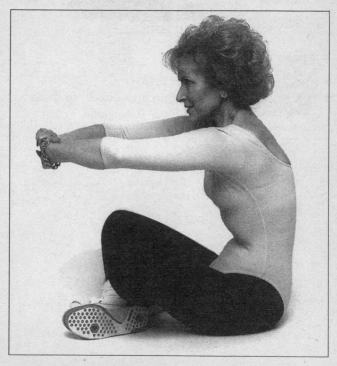

2 *Abdominal Stretch*

- Lie face down, supporting yourself on your forearms and elbows.
- Ease the shoulders upwards and back, and hold for 8–10 seconds.

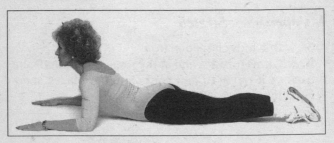

3 *Spine Stretch*

- Kneel, resting your hands in front.
- Pull your tummy in and arch the back upwards as much as possible. Hold for 8–10 seconds.

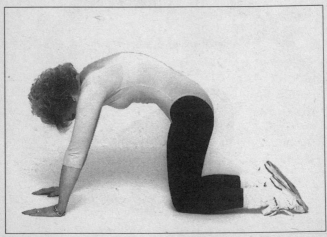

4 *Waist Stretch*

- Lie on your back with knees bent.
- Keeping the feet touching the floor, drop both knees over to one side. Hold for 8–10 seconds.
- Repeat to the other side.

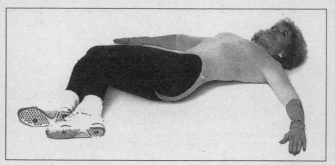

5 *Seat Stretch*

- Lie on your back with hands under your thighs.
- Squeeze the knees into your chest. Hold for 8–10 seconds.

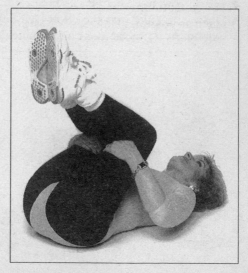

6 *Front Thigh Stretch*

- Lie face down with legs outstretched.
- Take hold of one foot and ease it towards your bottom, keeping the hips square and squeezing your buttocks. Hold for 8–10 seconds. Repeat with the other leg.

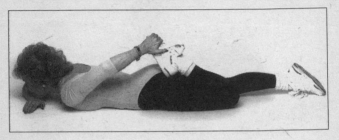

7 *Hamstring Stretch*

- Lie on your back with knees bent.
- Draw one knee into the chest (see below) and then extend the leg as far as is comfortable (see top of page

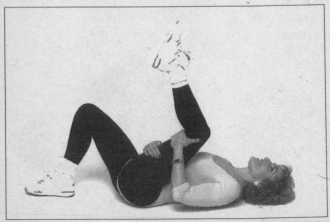

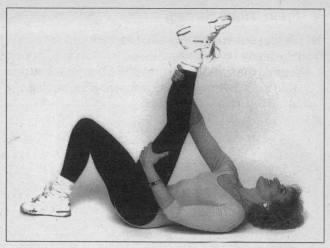

145), supporting the leg with your hands. Hold for 8–10 seconds before repeating with the other leg.

8 *Inner Thigh Stretch*

- Sit upright with soles of the feet together.
- Holding onto the ankles, ease the knees down towards the floor, pressing gently with the arms. Hold for 8–10 seconds.

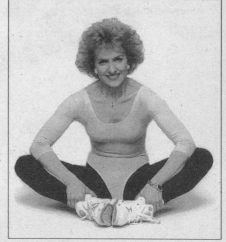

9 Outer Thigh Stretch

- Sit with your left leg extended in front and your right leg bent and crossed over it.
- Keeping your right hand on the floor, reach across with your left arm to ease the bent knee across the body. Hold for 8–10 seconds.
- Repeat with the other leg.

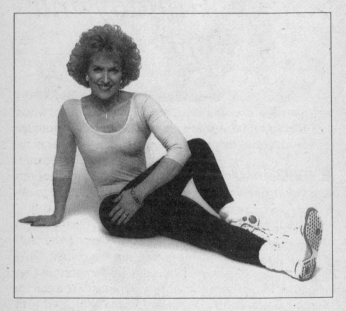

Ready, Steady... and Go On Holiday and Enjoy It!

So you've done it! You have stuck to the diet for 28 days and are now considerably slimmer than you were when you began. And if you've followed the exercise modules for five days a week and combined your aerobic activity with the toning exercises you will have a significantly slimmer, fitter and leaner body than you had a month ago. Give yourself a big pat on the back and enjoy packing your suitcase ready for the holiday of a lifetime.

There is a great psychological benefit in having a goal and a set length of time in which to gather together sufficient willpower to enable you to run the course. Now that your goal has been achieved it is so important that you don't let all that good work go to waste. You can try on your shorts and swimsuit and be really pleased with how you look compared with how you appeared 28 days ago. But, unless you are careful, you could easily undo a lot of the work that you have so industriously achieved.

When you go on holiday you have to make a decision. Are you going to eat as much as you can on the basis that you have paid for it so you are jolly well going to eat it – and consequently make yourself fat again? Or are you going to eat moderately and carefully and maintain this wonderful new body of yours? The choice is entirely up to you.

Over the last few weeks you have re-educated your palate and learnt which foods should be avoided and which ones are allowed on a low-fat diet. If you continue to follow these basic guidelines while you are on holiday, you should be able to maintain your new slim body. Gaining a pound or two won't matter, but it would be a real shame if you were to gain, say, seven pounds (3.2 kg). There is no need to deprive yourself and you certainly do not need to go hungry, but by choosing carefully from the menus that are offered to you, you really *can* maintain what you have achieved.

Don't get confused by the distinction between weight maintenance and weight loss. Many dieters fall into the trap of staying on a diet even after they have reached their goal weight. If you stay on a diet for too long, your metabolic rate will adjust to the new, lower level of eating and you won't lose any further weight, despite the fact that you are eating less than you did before you began the diet. The truth is you can eat a little more and still maintain your new weight. It has to be done carefully and should not involve eating vast quantities of forbidden foods. What you *can* do is eat a little more of the permitted foods you ate during the dieting period. If you follow this simple rule on holiday you should not regain your excess weight.

Here are my twenty tips for 'minimising the damage' while you are away. Follow these and you will keep any weight gain and loss of fitness to an absolute minimum.

1 Since your evening meal is likely to contain more than one course, eat only three meals a day.

2 Select your breakfast carefully, avoiding anything that is fried or spread with butter.

3 If you know you will be having a multi-course meal in the evening, try and keep lunch fairly light. Select a salad or fruit, and enjoy some local fresh bread – without butter of course!

4 For dinner, by all means eat five courses if they are offered, but ensure that the first course is really light such as melon, a fruit platter, or prawns – anything that is low in calories. For the second course choose clear soup in preference to one of the creamy alternatives and follow this with a sorbet or very light fish dish. The main course should be as free from fat as possible. Avoid anything that is deep-fried or cooked in butter or pastry. Eat as many vegetables as you like as long as they are cooked and served without butter. Don't be afraid to ask the waiter for your portion to be prepared without fat.

5 After the main course, select a dessert you enjoy, but again steer clear of cakes and anything cooked or served in pastry. Fresh fruit, meringue, a little ice cream, or fruit served in wine or liqueur are all delicious and should always be chosen in preference to high fat alternatives such as crème brûlée, soufflés, trifles or pies. Avoid cream and ask for a tiny portion of ice cream instead.

6 Do not be tempted by the cheese board. Since most hard cheeses contain in excess of 30 per cent fat, these are a real minefield for the dieter and should be avoided.

7 To finish off your evening meal, by all means have a petit four if you can select one that is virtually fat-free, e.g. a Chinese gooseberry dipped in icing sugar, or a piece of Turkish delight. Avoid the chocolates

and marzipan sweets. You can enjoy a cup of coffee but take it with milk not cream.

8 Throughout the day try to avoid between-meal snacks. The odd ice cream eaten between meals every day soon adds up, whereas if it is eaten as part of your snack lunch or dinner it will do minimal damage.

9 If you are going to be staying in a self-catering establishment in a country where dieting is not a high priority, then taking a low-calorie salad dressing away with you could be a real blessing.

10 Try to be as physically active as you possibly can each day of your holiday. Swim, run, play games, dance the night away – anything that will help to burn calories *and* keep your metabolic rate buoyant. The more active you are, the more food you can eat! There is no better way of working off a five-course dinner than to go dancing!

11 If you will be staying in a hotel complex which has its own gym, do take a pair of cushioned aerobic shoes and suitable clothing so that you can take full advantage of the facilities available.

12 Take this book to the beach and, if you have the confidence, repeat the body-toning exercises (pages 134 to 46). If the beach is too crowded and you don't want to make a spectacle of yourself, then do them in your hotel room or wherever you are staying. They will take only a few minutes a day and will help keep your muscles toned and make you feel better too.

13 If you make a conscious effort to be as active as possible, you will automatically tend to be careful about what you eat. You should not become a diet bore on holiday but, with a little careful thought, you can minimise any damage and enjoy the benefits.

14 If you do over-indulge one day, then try and be careful the next day to compensate. You will be pleasantly surprised how effective this is at keeping your weight under control, yet it will still allow you to enjoy the freedom and relaxation of the holiday environment. Compensating like this on alternate days should ensure you have a good time and will allow you to have treats that you may not indulge in at home.

15 It's never too late to get back on track. Even if you have over-indulged greatly over a couple of days, don't throw in the towel and feel that you have undone all the good that you did before you went away. Try to be more active and be cautious about what you eat for the next couple of days.

16 Since you are unlikely to have a pair of scales to hand while you are away, use a mirror to gauge your daily progress. Alternatively, take a tape measure with you, or try on the same skirt or pair of trousers every other day to monitor your size.

17 Clothes that don't fit too tightly will make you look slimmer, so bear this in mind when choosing outfits for your holiday. However, don't buy clothes that are *too* loose fitting, otherwise you might expand into them!

18 Having a tan can also make you appear slimmer, so for the first few days of your holiday you may find it worthwhile to apply some self-tanning lotion or leg make-up. Your local high street chemist should have a selection.

19 Remember, your family and friends have been tolerant of your campaign over the last four weeks. Don't spoil their holiday by being paranoid about your weight. Keep everything in perspective.

20 If you really do over-indulge while you are away, don't let it spoil your holiday, but do try and get back on the rails when you return by using the Beach Body Corrector Diet in the next section.

HAVE A WONDERFUL TIME!

STAGE 9

Beach Body Corrector Diet

If you have gained a few unwanted pounds (kg) on holiday, then by following this simple three-day diet you should hopefully be able to remove most of them.

Your daily allowance is ½ pint/10 fl oz (250 ml) skimmed or semi-skimmed milk and 5 fl oz (125 ml) unsweetened orange juice.

Do not eat between meals and try to stick strictly to the recommended menus for these three days. You will be surprised at how much weight you can reduce if you act promptly after your return from your holiday. From experience I know it works!

Try and be as active as possible and do 30 minutes' exercise each day for this three-day period to keep your metabolic rate as high as possible. It is worth making a few sacrifices while you are busily unpacking and getting your life back to normal again. Once you get over this short period of determined effort, you will be able to sit back and enjoy your new slim and fit body, which I hope you will maintain for good.

Do not follow the diet for longer than three days. To do so would reduce your metabolic rate which would be completely counterproductive. Likewise, do not return to the three-day diet too frequently as it will lose its effect.

DAY 1

Breakfast: 1 oz (25 g) any cereal with milk from allowance.

Lunch: Large salad with 3 oz (75 g) low-fat cottage cheese and fat-free dressing.

Dinner: 6 oz (150 g) white fish or 3 oz (75 g) red meat, served with 4 oz (100 g) jacket potato and unlimited vegetables.

DAY 2

Breakfast: Cut up ¼ melon and mix with 4 oz (100 g) strawberries. Top with 2 teaspoons diet yogurt.

Lunch: ½ pint/10 fl oz (250 ml) any clear soup, plus 1 slice (1 oz/25 g) toast, followed by 1 piece any fresh fruit.

Dinner: 4 oz (100 g) chicken (no skin), dry-fried with chopped peppers, onion, mushrooms, plus 1 oz (25 g) [dry weight] boiled rice mixed with 12 oz (300 g) tinned beansprouts. Serve with soy sauce.

DAY 3

Breakfast: 5 oz (125 g) diet yogurt plus 2 pieces any fresh fruit.

Lunch: 6 oz (150 g) jacket potato filled with 2 oz (50 g) cottage cheese and served with a large salad and a little fat-free dressing.

Dinner: 4 oz (100 g) chicken (no skin), served with unlimited green vegetables and carrots plus a little gravy, followed by 1 piece any fresh fruit.

STAGE 10

Maintaining Your New Weight

There are many benefits in following a low-fat diet. Not only do your tastebuds change (many people find the taste of fatty food becomes repulsive and indigestible), but your general feeling of wellbeing and your energy levels are increased to such an extent that you often feel significantly younger than your years. Add to this the fact that you look so much better after losing the unwanted fat from your body, well, it's like being a brand new person, and you don't want to lose that sense of feeling on top of the world.

Having achieved your goal it is obviously important to sustain it and, provided you don't slip back into your old, high-fat eating habits, this can be accomplished without too much difficulty. My simple golden rules for weight maintenance are as follows:

Ten Tips For Successful Weight Maintenance

1 Always select low-fat alternatives and check the nutrition panel to ascertain the fat content of foods *before* you buy them.

2 Continue to eat a low-fat diet and never add fat while preparing or serving food. However, you may now add a few more dressings to salads and occasionally eat a little, low-fat hard cheese.

3 Eat as much as you like of low-fat foods at meal times. Continue to eat three meals a day, but avoid between-meal snacks. Nibbling between meals can seriously damage your waistline.

4 Continue to exercise regularly. This will not only keep your heart fitter, but it will also help keep your metabolic rate higher so that weight maintenance becomes easier. It is important to find a form of exercise you enjoy.

5 Avoid temptation by not keeping biscuits and sweets (or, in fact, anything you think might tempt you in a weak moment) in the house. Instead, have plenty of fresh fruit available for you, your children and even the non-weight-conscious members of your family to consume. Also, fat-free cakes can soon become firm favourites with the family.

6 When dining out, enjoy yourself and by all means relax the rules a little, but try to be sensible when making your selection from the menu. It is easier to limit the damage than to cure the problem later.

7 Keep an eye on the scales and the tape measure. If you gain more than 2 lb (1 kg) in weight or more than

1 in (2.5 cm) at any circumference, return to the diet for two days and your weight should return to normal. It is a great deal easier to lose one or two pounds (kg) than three or four!

8 Never skip a meal as this can lead to uncontrolled eating later. Also, please remember that it is important to eat breakfast every day as this helps to kick-start your metabolism.

9 The occasional dietary indiscretion is not the end of the world, but do remember that one lapse can lead to another. Before you know where you are, you may find yourself on a slippery slope and returning to your old eating habits – the ones that made you over-weight in the first place – so indulge with caution!

10 Realise that weight maintenance is totally within your control. If you want to stay slim you can do so. Keep a 'before' photograph of yourself to hand, and each time you contemplate whether that cream cake really is worth it, look at that photograph.

Weight and Inch Loss Record Chart

Date:				
Weight				
Total weight lost to date				
Bust				
Waist				
Hips				
Widest part				
L. Thigh				
R. Thigh				
L. Knee				
R. Knee				
L. Arm				
R. Arm				
Total inches lost this week				
Total to date				

				Total loss

Index of Recipes

At Last –

A DIET AND FITNESS CLUB THAT COMBINES A HEALTHY LOW-FAT DIET WITH SAFE AND EFFECTIVE EXERCISE CLASSES

Rosemary Conley Diet and Fitness Clubs are the natural progression for a fitter, healthier lifestyle. Now you can follow Rosemary Conley's Hip and Thigh Diet in the company of others and benefit from weekly encouragement, advice and support.

Every class offers a weigh-in, presentation of a certificate to the 'Slimmer of the Week', followed by a 45-minute workout. Certificates are also awarded to everyone as they lose each stone in weight and a Certificate of Achievement when they reach their goal.

The classes are suitable for all fitness levels from beginners to advanced and, whether you have a little or a lot of weight to lose, our specially trained instructors will ensure you are made very welcome. You will receive all the help and encouragement that you need with the diet and the exercises.

All instructors are personally selected by Rosemary Conley and are trained to achieve the Royal Society of Arts Exercise To Music qualification in association with the Sports Council, and have also attended the Rosemary Conley Diet and Fitness Club Training Course.

For details of classes in your area call (0509) 620222.